Treatment Procedures in Communicative Disorders

Treatment Procedures in Communicative Disorders

M. N. HEGDE, PhD
California State University–Fresno

 COLLEGE-HILL PRESS, San Diego, California

College-Hill Press, Inc.
4284 41st Street
San Diego, California 92105

Library of Congress Cataloging in Publication Data
Main entry under title:

Hegde, M. N., 1941–
Treatment procedures in communicative disorders.

  Includes bibliographies and indexes.
  1. Speech, Disorders of—Treatment. 2. Language disorders—Treatment.
3. Speech therapy. 4. Communicative disorders—Treatment. I. Title.

RC423.H383 1985   616.85'506   85-14934

ISBN 0-88744-147-5

Printed in the United States of America

To Prema and Manu

CONTENTS

INTRODUCTION

This book is written for practicing speech-language pathologists and student clinicians in training programs. The main focus of the book is the treatment of communicative disorders. Generally speaking, treatments of different disorders are considered separately, with the implication that each disorder is treated in a unique manner. On the other hand, the approach taken in this book is that there are treatment principles and procedures that can be applied to all types of communicative disorders. This is not to suggest that the uniqueness of individuals or disorders should be ignored. On the contrary, the treatment model presented in this book seeks to clarify the issue of commonality and uniqueness. It is suggested that treatment principles are based on generality and procedures on uniqueness.

The book presents an integrated model of treatment in a single source. The model has its empirical bases, but it is not theoretical. A major purpose of the author is to describe techniques that clinicians can use in treating clients on a day-to-day basis. At the same time, every effort has been made to put the practical treatment procedures in the context of broader and empirically based scientific principles. The author believes that speech-language pathology, which is trying to broaden its scientific bases, cannot afford to take a cookbook approach to treatment. Nor can it afford to base treatment procedures upon rational arguments and logical assumptions that are not supported empirically.

The book emphasizes clinician accountability in terms of both legal and scientific requirements. Practical methods of documenting effectiveness of treatment and improvement in client behaviors are described. Strategies for documenting treatment effectiveness in individual clients without the aid of complex statistical techniques are summarized. It is well known that clinician accountability depends upon the measurement of client behaviors. Therefore, objective and verifiable procedures of measurement are described and emphasized throughout the book.

There are common principles of selecting target behaviors for training. These principles, along with suggestions on how to select multiple target behaviors, are offered. The importance of selecting target behaviors from the standpoint of long term maintenance is pointed out.

In the final analysis, a clinician's task is to increase certain desirable communicative behaviors in clients while decreasing certain undesirable and interfering behaviors. Therefore, in two chapters, basic techniques of increasing a variety of communicative behaviors, and those of decreasing undesirable behaviors, are specified. In a later chapter, a method for writing comprehensive treatment programs for clients with speech and language problems is given. In addition, the reasons for and procedures of making changes in written treatment programs are specified.

A significant clinical problem is the sequencing of treatment. A good program may be ineffective simply because of inappropriate sequencing of target behaviors. Before they are taught, many target behaviors must be simplified by identifying their smaller components that are learned relatively easily. Subsequently, the learned components must be integrated into the final target behavior. A related problem is presented by clients who just do not produce target behaviors at all. In such cases, the behaviors must be shaped into existence. Most clients in these situations need additional help in terms of modeling, instruction, prompting, and manual guidance. All of these techniques are described with examples.

One of the biggest clinical challenges faced by clinicians today is the maintenance of clinically learned behaviors. This problem has been conceptualized in terms of "generalization." It is possible, however, that the concepts and techniques associated with the term generalization are not appropriate for the clinical purposes of response maintenance. Some of these conceptual and methodological problems are discussed along with several techniques designed to achieve response maintenance.

It is hoped that practicing as well as student clinicians will find this book useful in planning and executing treatment programs for their clients. It is also hoped that the book will help clinicians plan treatment programs on the basis of scientific and professional principles. These principles are a basis for designing flexible treatment programs that can be modified to suit individual clients with a variety of communicative disorders. The principles and procedures described in the book seek to fulfill legal, professional, and scientific demands made upon speech-language pathologists.

Chapter 1

A Treatment Paradigm for Communicative Disorders

In Chapter 1, the following points will be discussed:

- A treatment paradigm for communicative disorders
- Treatment principles and procedures
- Contingencies as treatment variables
- Logical versus empirical validity
- Treatment targets versus treatment procedures
- Treatment programs versus treatment variables
- Some legal considerations (PL 94-142) and individual educational plans (IEPs)

Discussions of treatment techniques in communicative disorders tend to be disorder specific. Most textbooks typically describe treatment of different communicative disorders separately. Clinicians who seek information on treatment procedures also tend to be concerned about specific disorders. Beginning clinicians often believe that each disorder of communication is treated with unique techniques. Such a belief is understandable in light of the way most university curricula are organized. Students typically take separate courses on disorders, such as language, articulation, or stuttering. Each academic course necessarily focuses upon the unique characteristics of a given disorder. As a result, the treatment procedures offered in academic courses also tend to focus upon the unique aspects of treating given disorders.

The belief that different disorders are treated entirely differently may be further strengthened by the medical model that is often used in describing and assessing communicative disorders. Disorders are often described in terms of "diagnostic categories." In the assessment of communicative disorders, considerable emphasis is placed upon "differential diagnosis." In medicine, treatment is typically directed toward the original cause of physical diseases. Therefore, diagnosis, which is the detection of the causes of particular diseases, is especially important. When different causes of different disorders are determined, they are treated differently.

An uncritical application of this model to the assessment and treatment of communicative disorders can create the impression that each speech and language problem is treated by totally unique procedures. In communicative disorders, differential diagnosis often amounts to differential descriptions of disorders, not the detection of different causes. Furthermore, disorders are described in terms of client behaviors. For example, a disorder of articulation may be described in terms of the production of various speech sounds, whereas stuttering may be described in terms of dysfluency forms and frequencies. Similarly, the descriptions of a language problem differ from those of a voice problem.

The fact that most communicative disorders take different response forms does not necessarily mean that their treatment procedures do not share common features. A closer examination of treatment procedures applied to various disorders of communication reveals many common treatment elements. At the same time, the treatment of given individuals and disorders may include some unique features. In order to find out the treatment aspects that are common across disorders and clients and those that are unique, a distinction must be made between treatment principles and treatment procedures.

TREATMENT PRINCIPLES AND PROCEDURES

Both clinical and nonclinical behavioral research has shown that individuals share common characteristics while still being unique in many respects. Commonality exists because of similarities between disorders and people who exhibit them. Uniqueness is a result of special response characteristics of given disorders and unusual histories of individual clients.

Some unique aspects of treatment are indeed based upon the special response characteristics of particular disorders. In some ways, techniques designed to evoke the correct production of /s/ is different from those evoking the preposition *on*. Even then, the differences are not absolute. Different response evocation techniques themselves share common elements. For example, modeling or verbal instructions may be common across these techniques.

It is generally believed that the uniqueness of treatment procedures stems from differential diagnosis of various disorders. A more important reason for some unique aspects of treatment may be those factors that make each individual unique. In other words, different procedures may be necessary in treating the same disorder across individuals. For example, all clients with a specific language disorder may not react positively to the same type of stimulus conditions or response consequences. All stutterers may not react the same way to the same reinforcers or punishers. Therefore, some unique aspects of treatment are a result of the unusual personal histories brought to the training situation.

It is evident that commonality and uniqueness are both real. In essence, the basic principles of treatment are common, whereas certain specifics of treatment procedures are unique to disorders, clients, or both. Treatment principles can be defined as empirical rules from which treatment procedures are derived. A clinician who knows a principle can derive a variety of procedures from it. Treatment principles are a product of controlled experimental research. Ideally, the principles should be based on replicated research with a certain degree of generality. As such, accepted principles should be reliable, valid, and comprehensive. When such principles are formulated, it should be possible to derive different treatment procedures from them. These procedures can then be used with different disorders, clients, and in different situations.

Treatment procedures can be defined as the technical operations the clinician performs in order to effect changes in client behaviors. In the final analysis, treatment procedures refer to certain clinician actions. These actions induce changes in a client's communicative behaviors. In a later section it will be shown that most clinician actions are typically performed before and after an attempted response on the part of the client.

Broad Principles and Specific Procedures

While treatment principles are relatively broad and general, the treatment procedures are typically specific to a given disorder or client. For example, the statement that certain consequences, when made contingent upon a behavior, increase the rate of that behavior is a principle. It is the well-known principle of positive reinforcement. There is enough empirical evidence to suggest that the principle applies to different people, different age groups, and even members of different species. In other words, the principle has some generality, and therefore, it amounts to an empirical rule.

In the actual application of the principle of positive reinforcement, the clinician must derive some specific procedures that suit the individual client, the disorder being treated, or both. The principle does not specify what particular thing or event will reinforce a given response in a given client. That is a matter of particular procedures; the clinician will have to find out. For example, a clinician might determine that a given client's correct production of /s/ can be reinforced by verbal praise. The clinician might also find out that the correct production of the same phoneme in another client cannot be reinforced by verbal praise alone, but that tokens backed up by 2 minutes of play activity can. Each of these cases illustrates a client-specific procedure of treatment derived from the principle of positive reinforcement.

There are a number of treatment principles. In addition to the principle of positive reinforcement, there are principles such as negative reinforcement, extinction, punishment, discrimination, generalization and stimulus control. Most of these principles were originally formulated on the basis of extensive laboratory research across species. Subsequently, in applied behavioral analysis, these principles have been shown to be reliable and valid. In the field of communicative disorders, many successful treatment procedures have been derived from these and other principles. In later chapters, each of these principles will be described, and a variety of specific procedures that have been derived from them will be illustrated.

Fewer Principles, Many Procedures

It is possible to derive a variety of treatment procedures from a single treatment principle. The principle of positive reinforcement, for example, has given rise to a variety of specific reinforcement procedures including primary reinforcers, verbal reinforcers, conditioned generalized reinforcers, informative feedback, and so on. Similarly, the principles of punishment and extinction have generated multiple procedures to achieve reductions in response rates. As such, principles are fewer than procedures.

It is important to understand the principles of treatment. The clinician who does not understand treatment principles may have to search for procedures every time a new client is encountered. A distinction between a professional and a technician can often be made on this basis. A professional understands the principles, whereas a technician understands only the procedures that were presented to him or her. If abstract treatment principles are absent, new clients, disorders, and clinical settings may be baffling. An understanding of treatment principles makes it possible to design flexible treatment plans.

Procedures without principles can be rigid prescriptions that are hard to modify in order to suit individual clients or disorders. Such procedures are often a part of "cookbooks" of "treatment." A professional discipline cannot make significant progress without underlying treatment principles that are based upon experimental evidence.

Abstract Principles, Concrete Procedures

Another distinction between treatment principles and procedures is that the former are abstract and conceptual, whereas the latter are concrete, practical, and measurable. Principles are the conceptual bases of practical treatment techniques. Fully validated principles are summary statements of experimental evidence. At a conceptual level, the principles describe relations between events. Abstract statements that constitute principles are based upon different kinds of experimental evidence. For example, the principle of punishment is based upon a variety of specific experiments involving different kinds of stimuli, intensities of those stimuli, correlation of those stimuli with other kinds of stimuli, manner of their introduction, and so on. These different kinds of experimental observations are abstracted into the principle of punishment. It simply specifies that certain stimulus events, when made contingent upon a response, can decrease the rate of that response.

An abstract principle suggests practical methods that can be applied in treatment. In deriving procedures from a principle, the clinician often has to go back to the specific experimental manipulations on which the principle was based. To take the example of punishment again, the clinician may have to look at particular kinds of stimuli that were indeed used in the original experiments to identify tentative stimuli that have the potential of acting as punishers.

Unlike treatment principles, the procedures are specified in operational (measurable) terms. Unless the procedures specify what the clinician should do, they cannot be applied in practical situations. Procedures that are not concrete cannot be replicated by other clinicians. Operationally defined procedures make it possible to measure the effectiveness of treatment and thereby document clinician accountability.

A TREATMENT PARADIGM
FOR COMMUNICATIVE DISORDERS

In order to understand the philosophical bases of principles and procedures of treatment better, it is necessary to take a look at the treatment paradigm. A treatment paradigm can be defined as an overall philosophical position concerning the subject matter (communicative behaviors) and how to modify disorders thereof. The paradigm can be described in terms of its conceptual and procedural bases.

The Conceptual Bases of the Paradigm

The paradigm presented in this book is based on the position that for the most part, the behaviors the speech-language clinician deals with are a function of two kinds of contingencies. A contingency describes an interdependent relation between certain variables. One kind of contingency involves genetic or neurophysiological variables, whereas the other kind involves environmental variables. In other words, there are interdependent neurophysiological or genetic variables and interdependent environmental variables that determine behaviors. More importantly, the two sets of variables themselves are interdependent, creating a more complex contingency. According to the paradigm, practically all of our behaviors, including communicative behaviors and disorders, are determined by this complex contingency.

Research into neurophysiological or genetic contingencies that partially control communicative behaviors and disorders have become more and more sophisticated in recent years. It is well known that an intact neurophysiological mechanism is necessary for the normal acquisition of speech and language behaviors. Differences in the organization or functioning of neurophysiological mechanisms can affect the way communicative behaviors are acquired or maintained. The importance of genetic mechanisms in the etiology of several speech and language disorders has also been researched in recent years. From a clinical standpoint, neurophysiological and genetic factors may restrict the rate or scope of improvement that can be obtained by treatment. They may also partly determine the amount or type of treatment needed.

Sophisticated research on how genetic or neurophysiological mechanisms affect treatment considerations has barely begun, however. Much of the available genetic and neurophysiological information concerning communicative disorders cannot be effectively used in the treatment process. It is hoped that in the near future more will be learned about integrating this type of information with treatment considerations.

Manipulable Environmental Contingencies. In the treatment of communicative disorders, environmental contingencies can be currently manipulated more successfully than organic contingencies. This is also true of those communicative disorders that are often described as neurologically or organically based. In dealing with either an aphasic patient or a child with a surgically repaired cleft, the task of the speech-language clinician is to modify the client's communicative behaviors, using certain environmental manipulations. Currently, there is no direct access to those organic contingencies that create disorders of communication. For example, various genetic conditions that are associated with syndromes of language disorders cannot be altered directly. Similarly, brain damage that results from a cerebrovascular accident cannot be altered in order to eliminate aphasia.

Some of the organic conditions that can be manipulated (such as the surgical repair of cleft palate) are handled by the medical profession. However, such manipulations are usually not sufficient to fully alter the communicative disorders associated with the original organic deficit. After the organic manipulations have been done, the speech-language clinician then has to modify the communicative behaviors. The techniques available to the clinician for doing so are typically environmental.

Since the manipulable environmental contingencies are the treatment procedures, the nature of such contingencies must be fully understood. Environmental contingencies can be defined as three sets of interdependent variables that correspond to stimuli, responses, and consequences. As soon as some target behaviors are identified for a given client, the clinician usually proceeds to arrange certain stimulus conditions for those behaviors. In order to do this, pictures, real objects, and questions that might evoke the responses may be selected. The clinician might plan on modeling the target behaviors so that the client can imitate them. Later on in the training sequence, prompts may be used to evoke the correct responses from the client. All of these stimulus conditions are antecedents of target behaviors. They are presented before the responses are expected.

Typically, the correct responses expected of the client are predetermined. Technically speaking, the topograpical aspects of responses are specified to the client. Modeling the correct response is a way of specifying the response topography that will be accepted. As soon as the client responds in some way to the stimuli presented (including modeling), the clinician usually makes a judgment as to whether the response is acceptable. If it is, the clinician responds in one manner, and if it is not, in a different manner. If the client did not respond at all, the clinician might react still differently. These clinician reactions are the consequences of the client behaviors. Some kinds of consequences create new behaviors or increase the frequency of current behaviors, while others make existing behaviors less probable in the future.

All of the client and the clinician behaviors can be succinctly described in terms of a contingency. What the clinician does has an effect on what the client does, and client behaviors determine the consequences, which are indeed the clinician responses. In essence, the stimulus conditions, the client response characteristics, and the consequences the clinician arranges for those responses are the three interrelated variables in a contingency.

Based on the Concepts and Methods of Science. Another conceptual basis of the treatment paradigm is the philosophy of science. The paradigm dictates that all concepts and procedures used within its scope be empirically validated. There is very little room for clinical or theoretical speculation. Speculative concepts are usually not of much help to a practicing clinician. It would be difficult to base effective treatment procedures on a paradigm that simply assumes a lot about the disorders that need to be treated. In order to be useful, the treatment paradigm should stay very close to empirical evidence. Cause-and-effect relations must be demonstrated, not just assumed. They should be demonstrated through experimental research in which the causal variables were actually manipulated by the researcher. This type of research is more fully described in Chapter 3.

Much of the clinical controversies and apparent treatment diversities are due to the predominance of nonexperimental research in speech-language pathology. Nonexperimental research tends to encourage theoretical speculation, which in turn leads to fruitless controversies. Untested treatment procedures may be offered and vigorously advocated by different clinicians. Often, treatment procedures are offered by pure theoreticians who may not have an opportunity to verify their own suggestions. Suggestions of this kind have sometimes come from experts in the field of linguistics. Despite the fact that such clinical procedures or suggestions for treatment were never experimentally verified, they may stay on the books only to confuse clinicians.

The Procedural Bases of the Paradigm

The treatment paradigm offered in this book leads to procedures that can be readily applied in the treatment of communicative disorders. Ideally, treatment procedures should be objective, measurable, replicable, and empirical. Methods that would help document the effectiveness of treatment should be an integral part of the procedures. These requirements stem from scientific, legal, and social considerations.

Response Rates as Target Behaviors. The paradigm suggests that observable rate of client responses be the treatment targets. The client responses are also known as the dependent variables, and when they are observable behaviors, they can be verified by other clinicians. Communicative behaviors are most observable when described in terms of response rates of speakers. The speaking behaviors can be broken down into specific responses that can be counted in real numbers. For example, how many times a child produced the grammatic morpheme *ing* in a ten-minute conversational speech can be specified in actual numbers. Similarly, the number of words or parts of words repeated, the number of times a given phoneme was produced correctly, the duration for which a given vocal pitch was sustained, or the number of manual signs a deaf individual produced can be measured relatively precisely.

There are measures other than the rate of responses, and clinicians have often used them. The rating scales are an excellent example of popular measures not based on real numbers. Disorders may be rated as mild, moderate, or severe, and such ratings may be considered "measurement" of communicative behaviors. Each judgmental category may also be assigned a number, such as 3, 5, and 7. Rating scales, however, offer no direct and meaningful measures of specific behaviors. One would not know the actual number of times a given behavior was produced. Instead of saying that a person was a "severe" stutterer with a rating scale value of 7, one might more precisely say that the person exhibited dysfluencies or stutterings on 13 (or whatever) per cent of the words spoken. The reader, if desired, can make his or her own judgments regarding the "severity" based upon the reported amounts of stuttering.

Rate of responses, measured in real numbers, can make it possible for other observers to verify treatment gains or changes in client behaviors. Other observers can count the same behaviors in the same client and see if the values arrived at agree with those of the clinician. Objectivity in clinical activity is achieved when a given clinician's measures can be verified by other clinicians. In other words, agreement among different observers (clinicians) constitutes objectivity.

A potential problem with agreement among observers is that it may not be based upon measurement. One might find plenty of agreement at the level of opinions held by different clinicians, which may or may not enhance objectivity. In some cases, such opinions may be totally invalid.

Communicative behaviors described in terms of presumed mental, cognitive, or neurophysiological processes are hard to measure and verify objectively. Such internal processes presumed to take place within individuals are theoretically based, and are often not observed directly. For example, a target behavior in a language training program might be defined either as linguistic competence or as production of specified grammatic morphemes, or vocabulary items (words). The former is an inferred entity, whereas the latter two are observable. In Chapter 3, selection and definition of target behaviors will be discussed more fully.

Measurable Treatment Procedures. Another methodological basis of the treatment paradigm is that the treatment techniques used must be replicable. The treatment program may be repeated by the same clinician with different clients. On the other hand, different clinicians may use the same procedure with their clients in different settings. Such replications help establish generality of treatment techniques. In addition, replications are useful in determining whether a treatment procedure can be effective with other clients in new settings when used by different clinicians. In that process, the kinds of changes that enhance treatment effects may also be determined.

Treatment techniques described in vague and nonmeasurable terms do not lend themselves to replication. If it is not clear how a given technique was used, then it cannot be repeated.

Logical Versus Empirical Validity. Finally, treatment procedures should be empirical, in the sense that their effects are demonstrated in actual experience. When clinicians read about different treatment techniques that often conflict with each other, they may find them equally appealing, rational, and plausible. In other words, most treatment procedures appear logical. However, the clinician needs to make a distinction between logical and empirical validity. What is logically valid may or may not be empirically valid, although empirical validity usually assures logical validity.

Statements that are mutually consistent and do not violate rules of logic have logical validity. But those statements may turn out to be invalid in actual experiments or in clinical treatment situations. For example, there is nothing illogical in the suggestion that lack of parental affection causes language delay in a child, or that psychosexual repressions and regressions result in stuttering. However, when parents show affection in the absence of verbal exchange, the child may not learn language, thus showing that the logical statement did not have empirical validity. Similarly, a treatment based exclusively on the theory of psychosexual aberrations may not reduce stuttering.

Clinicians need procedures that go beyond logical validity. In speech-language pathology, "new" treatment programs are sometimes offered simply on the basis of logical validity. As pointed out earlier, if research clinicians refrain from offering treatment suggestions that are not experimentally verified, a lot of controversy and confusion can be avoided.

TREATMENT TARGETS
VERSUS TREATMENT PROCEDURES

In clinical literature, there is sometimes a confusion between treatment targets and treatment techniques. It is true that a comprehensive treatment program would include a description of both. At the same time, it is necessary to distinguish treatment targets from procedures, since that distinction is important from conceptual and technical standpoints.

Treatment targets are client behaviors, whereas the procedures are mostly clinician behaviors. In other words, what the client is expected to do is the target, and what the clinician does is the treatment. This simple and rather obvious rule is sometimes violated when a treatment technique is identified in terms of a target behavior.

Examples of confusion between treatment targets and procedures abound in speech and language pathology. A new stuttering treatment may be described as the "airflow" technique, or a new language treatment may be described as "cognitive reorganization." But the "airflow" refers to what the stutterer is expected to do, and hence is a treatment target, not a procedure. A treatment procedure exists only when the clinician actions necessary to teach appropriate airflow management are specified. Similarly, cognitive reorganization is not what the clinician does; it is what is presumed to take place within the client. The treatment would be the procedures by which cognitive reorganization is achieved, if at all. Similarly, in the area of articulation, "phonologic rules" do not refer to treatment procedures. Such rules are simply supposed to underlie observed regularities in response patterns. How such rules are taught (if they are) might constitute a treatment technique.

It is quite possible that not as many treatment procedures exist as may be supposed. Different treatment procedures may simply involve different target behaviors. Some target behaviors may be more useful than others. Certain target behaviors may improve the overall communicative skills better than certain other behaviors. It is therefore natural that clinicians keep looking for new target behaviors that are most effective in improving the quality of the client's verbal behavior. It does not mean that new treatment techniques are being invented at the same time, however.

Take, for instance, the theoretical shifts in the areas of language and articulation. During the early days of language intervention, clinicians had often focused exclusively upon vocabulary training. Subsequently, the emphasis was shifted to the training of various syntactic and morphologic aspects of language. Later on, for a brief time, the emphasis was on training semantic concepts. In more recent years, clinicians have been asked to train pragmatic functions or rules. In the treatment of articulation disorders, emphasis has been shifted from single phoneme training to distinctive features, and again to phonologic rules or processes.

It is important to realize that when the answer to the question "what to train" during language or articulation therapy was being shifted around, new treatment procedures were hardly invented. Different methods of analyzing language and articulation did not produce new treatment procedures. What were new at any given time were the target behaviors or, perhaps, a new terminology to describe the old target behaviors. New procedures to train those new or redefined behaviors were hardly presented. Many times, the question of how to train those behaviors was not addressed at all.

Lack of a clear distinction between target behaviors and treatment procedures may be responsible for poor descriptions of treatment techniques in many treatment programs. Apparently, many clinicians assume that when they describe a new treatment target, they have automatically suggested a new treatment procedure. Much worse, some clinicians do not see a need to describe their treatment procedures at all; they describe only their target behaviors.

As indicated earlier, a treatment technique should specify what the clinician ought to do in order to achieve the treatment target. When this is done, what emerges is a description of the stimulus conditions the clinician needs to arrange, and the kinds of feedback that must be provided to the client under the differing conditions of correct, incorrect, and lack of responses. In other words, the concept of a contingency will become clear. The treatment paradigm described in this book suggests that contingencies are the treatment variables in communicative disorders. Those contingencies can be placed on any kind of empirically valid target behavior.

TREATMENT PROGRAMS AND TREATMENT VARIABLES

The term treatment program, as used in this book, is an overall description of target behaviors, treatment variables, measurement procedures, generalization and maintenance strategies, parent training or counseling, follow-up, booster treatment, and so on. As such, a program is a comprehensive plan of action that includes different kinds of clinical activities designed to achieve certain overall objectives. Essentially, a treatment program describes all of the clinician and client behaviors.

Treatment variables, on the other hand, refer to technical operations performed by the clinician in order to induce, modify, or eliminate certain client behaviors. Treatment variables are also known as independent variables, which may include certain stimulus manipulations such as modeling. More importantly, they include consequences programmed for target behaviors. What the clinician does after having observed a correct, incorrect, or lack of response constitutes the programmed consequence. Therefore, only a portion of a treatment program will be concerned with treatment variables. In this book, terms such as treatment variables, treatment techniques, and training procedures will refer to the clinician's manipulations of independent variables, including stimulus conditions and response consequences. The term treatment program, on the other hand, will be used in the broader sense to include an overall clinical strategy.

SOME LEGAL CONSIDERATIONS (PL 94-142)

It is well known that Public Law 94-142 mandates clinical and educational services to school-age children who need them. The law has had a significant impact on the delivery of special educational programs, including speech-language services in public schools. The United States Congress passed the bill and it was signed into law in 1975. The law took effect in three stages, starting in October 1977. During its first phase, the law required that each state government begin the development of a comprehensive program for the education of all handicapped children. Perhaps the most important requirement under the law was that for each child in need of special educational services, an individual educational plan (IEP) be developed. In addition, the law required that the rights and the confidentiality of the child and the family be protected, and that parents be involved in the execution of the special educational programs designed for their children.

During its second phase, which went into effect in 1978, the scope of the law covered all handicapped children between 3 and 18 years of age. It also required each state government to submit revised annual plans specifying its special educational programs. The last phase went into effect in 1980 and covered children between 3 and 21 years of age. In general, the law specifies that initially each handicapped child must be assessed to determine the type and extent of the problem. The assessment should include multiple and nondiscriminatory tools. Each child should have access to free and public education designed to suit his or her special needs. The handicapped child should be placed in the least restrictive environment, and whenever possible, the child should be mainstreamed. Finally, needed supplementary services should be provided. It is not the purpose of this chapter to review the full scope of the law. The reader should consult other sources (Arena, 1978; Lerner, Dawson, and Horvath, 1980).

From the standpoint of developing clinical speech and language programs, the IEP guidelines are important. In essence, an IEP describes an educational program specific to a given child. Based on the assessment results, the IEP will contain statements concerning the child's current communicative behaviors. It will then specify the target behaviors in operational terms, procedures to achieve them, the date the program will be initiated, predicted duration of the program, and the objective criteria to be used in judging the success of the program. How often the evaluative criteria will be applied should also be specified. Under the law, the effects of the program should be evaluated at least once a year. The entire program should be developed as a team effort involving the educational agency, teachers, parents, and other professionals. Whenever it is needed and considered appropriate, the child may also participate in the process of treatment planning.

Although an IEP is required under the law, it is not a legal contract. The clinicians should consider the development of an IEP a scientific and professional task. The clinician working in the public schools is certainly bound by the requirements of the law. But it is a mistake to think that what the law requires is merely a matter of governmental and administrative bureaucracy, which it often is. Many of the requirements of the law are also the requirements of the philosophy and methodology of science.

It must also be realized that what the law asks clinicians to do does not take away the aspect of clinical judgment based on scientific facts and observations. Selection of target behaviors, development of treatment procedures, documentation of the effectiveness of treatment or changes in the client behaviors, and specification of evaluative criteria are all a matter of scientific and professional judgment. For example, exactly when the treatment program will be completed by a given child is stated not in terms of certainty, but in terms of probability, which reflects the best clinical judgment. It is a scientific statement, not a legal promise. When the child will actually complete the program will depend upon a number of uncontrolled factors, including the child's rate of learning, the family's cooperation, the frequency and duration of treatment sessions, the severity of the disorder being treated, and many others. From the professional standpoint, the treatment program will be terminated only when the target behaviors are learned and maintained.

It is often thought that one of the most important effects of the law is to make the clinician more accountable. In other words, clinicians have to demonstrate objectively that under the treatment program, the client behaviors changed systematically. Subjective statements such as "the child has improved tremendously" or "has benefited from the services" are not acceptable when they are not substantiated by objective data. In addition, the target behaviors must be defined in measurable terms, so that changes in the frequency of those behaviors can be documented. It should be noted, however, that the need for legal mandates in matters such as these is somewhat ironic. Science has always required that the target behaviors be measurable, the procedures be specific, and the treatment effects be measured in terms of changes in the frequency of those behaviors. Scientifically oriented clinicians have always done these things, but unfortunately, the scientific foundations of our profession have not been as strong in the past as they are now.

The behavioral treatment paradigm presented in this chapter, and elaborated on throughout the book, antedates the legal requirements but is in full compliance with them. The treatment paradigm considers each individual as unique and requires that the individual behaviors be objectively measured. There is not much emphasis on evaluating the individual's behaviors in relation to group performance. The paradigm suggests that the target behaviors selected for clinical training be appropriate and useful to the particular client. It requires that the treatment procedure be described in objective and specific terms so that it can be replicated by other clinicians. There is a great deal of emphasis on documenting the effectiveness of treatment. In the coming chapters, many of these issues and procedures will be discussed in some detail.

SUMMARY

Some aspects of treatment are common across disorders and clients and some are unique. The treatment principles are common, whereas certain procedures can be unique.

Treatment principles are data-based empirical rules that are conceptual, relatively broad, and abstract. The treatment procedures are clinical operations derived from those principles. The procedures are many, and they are more specific than the principles.

A paradigm is an overall philosophical position concerning a subject matter. A treatment paradigm is a philosophy of treatment, based on the methods of science. The paradigm presented in the book suggests that a management of the contingency between stimulus, response, and consequence variables constitutes treatment.

In communicative disorders, currently manipulable contingencies are environmental. The contingency includes measurable response rates as target behaviors.

Logical validity is assumed when statements are internally consistent and do not violate the rules of logic. In contrast, empirical validity is assumed only when statements are based upon research evidence. Statements that are logically valid can be empirically false.

Treatment targets are client behaviors, whereas the treatment procedures are clinician behaviors.

A treatment program is an overall clinical strategy. Treatment variables are technical operations performed by the clinician.

Public Law 94-142 mandates clinical or special educational services to handicapped school-age children. Among other things, the law requires that an individual treatment plan be developed for each child and the treatment effects be documented objectively.

STUDY GUIDE

Answer the following questions in technical terms. Check your answers with the text. When necessary, rewrite your answers.

1. Why do some clinicians tend to believe that different disorders are treated differently?
2. Define treatment principles.
3. Define treatment procedures.
4. Give examples of treatment principles.
5. Give examples of treatment procedures.
6. Compare and contrast treatment principles and procedures.
7. What is a treatment paradigm?
8. What are the conceptual bases of the paradigm?
9. What are the procedural bases of the paradigm?
10. Define a contingency.
11. What are the two kinds of contingencies?

12. What kinds of contingencies are manipulable?
13. What are antecedents of behaviors?
14. What are consequences of behaviors?
15. Define replication.
16. What is objectivity?
17. What is empirical validity?
18. What is logical validity?
19. Are all logically valid statements empirically valid?
20. What kinds of research encourage speculation and fruitless controversy?
21. Distinguish between treatment targets and treatment procedures.
22. What is PL 94-142?
23. What are the requirements under PL 94-142 that affect clinical speech-language services in the public schools?
24. How does the treatment paradigm relate to the legal requirements of the law?
25. What are IEPs?
26. What do you understand by "multiple evaluative criteria"?
27. Are IEPs legal contracts?
28. How do you state when a treatment program will be terminated?
29. Describe the three phases of PL 94-142.
30. What are "nondiscriminatory tools of assessment"?

REFERENCES

Arena, J. (1978). *How to write an I.E.P.* Novato, CA: Academic Therapy Publications.

Lerner, J., Dawson, D., and Horvath, L. (1980). *Cases in learning and behavior problems: A guide to individualized education programs.* Boston: Houghton Mifflin.

Chapter 2

Documenting Treatment Effectiveness

In Chapter 1, a treatment paradigm, along with treatment principles and procedures, was described.

In Chapter 2, the following points will be described:

- Clinician accountability
- Improvement versus effectiveness
- Some basic concepts of science
- Similarities between scientific and clinical activity
- Need to document treatment effectiveness
- Two strategies for establishing treatment effectiveness
- Generality of treatment effects
- Selection of treatment techniques

In recent years, the issue of clinician accountability has received much public and professional attention. This is partly because of Public Law 94-142. As pointed out in Chapter 1, the law requires objective documentation of the effectiveness of special educational services rendered in public schools. Understandably, society will not continue to support services whose effects are questionable or are based upon subjective evaluations. The spirit of the law, however, extends beyond the public school settings. Professional services rendered anywhere should be justifiable on objective grounds.

Independent of legal requirements, there is a growing recognition among speech-language pathologists of a need to strengthen the scientific basis of clinical activities (Costello, 1979; Minifie, 1983; Ringel, 1972; Ringel, Trachtman, and Prutting, 1984; Zimmermann, 1984). If speech-language pathologists are to gain better public recognition as a scientific profession, they need to operate within the framework of science and its methodology. The education of speech-language pathologists should include a thorough understanding of the philosophy and methodology of science. This is probably an area in which clinicians are undertrained. Many graduates in communicative disorders may not have had significant course work in scientific concepts, philosophies, and methodologies.

Some stereotypic concepts of science may have had a negative impact on the education of speech-language pathologists. There is an implicit belief that "science" within the profession is restricted to certain subject matters such as anatomy, physiology, neurology, and acoustics. Study of language, articulation, stuttering, and so on may not be very "scientific." A related belief is that if it is desirable for a certain subject matter to be recognized as a branch of science, then all that must be done is to add the word "science" or "-ology" to it. Thus, empty phrases like "language science" and "aphasiology" have been created. Unfortunately, under the relabeled subject matter, research and writing may continue to be just as speculative and nonexperimental as before.

Science is no particular subject matter. It is not to be defined as physics, neurology, acoustics, or anatomy. Science is a certain philosophy, a particular disposition, and a set of methods. When those who study a given subject matter adopt that philosophy, learn those dispositions, and use those methods, they have a branch of science. In other words, how a subject matter is approached and studied will determine whether it is a science or not.

SCIENCE AS A PHILOSOPHY

In the final analysis, science amounts to a certain philosophy. It takes a unique approach to the study of the nature and events, including human affairs. As a philosophy, science believes in determinism. Determinism states that nothing happens without a cause. Events are determined (caused) by prior events, and it is possible to analyze those prior events. In behavioral sciences, events (behaviors) may also be determined by their consequences. Established behaviors may be a function of (determined by) both antecedent and consequent events. Extended to communicative disorders, the philosophy of science would assert that all communicative behaviors and their disorders have antecedent and consequent events that partly determine those behaviors and disorders.

As a philosophy, science believes in understanding, predicting, and controlling phenomena (Bachrach, 1969). It is often said that understanding, predicting, and controlling phenomena are the goals of science. We understand an event when we know what caused it. When we analyze cause-and-effect relations, we see patterns where before we had only seen some random happenings. When we understand the causes of events, we can predict them. Also, when causes are known, the effects can be modified. When scientists are able to modify a phenomenon, they will have gained control over it. Some of the similarities between this philosophy of science and that of clinical professions will be discussed in a later section.

SCIENCE AS A DISPOSITION

Science requires a certain disposition on the part of those who practice it (Bachrach, 1969; Skinner, 1953). Scientists tend to behave in ways that may be unique to them. It can even be said that science is essentially what scientists do. Scientists' behaviors shape science, and the products of science are also the products of their behaviors.

Scientists value evidence more than opinions, and objective demonstrations more than subjective statements. A scientist believes that it is the subject matter that knows best, not any person—including himself or herself (Skinner, 1953). Scientists tend to accept evidence, not authorities. Even though they have their feelings and opinions about the nature and causes of events, they are always willing to have them replaced by what has been experimentally demonstrated. Scientists are inclined to go without an explanation rather than accept one that is not based upon experimental evidence.

SCIENCE AS METHODS AND PROCEDURES

Science is a set of methods and procedures; probably this definition is better known than science as a disposition and as a philosophy. The methods and procedures of science are rules that dictate the activities of a scientist. Scientists are usually careful not to violate those rules. It is necessary to briefly review some of the basic procedures of science. A knowledge of those procedures is essential for establishing clinician accountability.

Scientific procedures suggest appropriate ways of answering research questions. The procedures dictate structures within which investigations can be conducted. Basically, the procedures of science are objective, by which it is meant that they and their results are publicly verifiable. The procedures are based on measurement. Unless phenomena are measured in objective ways, no further scientific operations can be performed on them. Such objective and measurement-based procedures make it possible to (1) manipulate variables and (2) establish cause-and-effect relations between events.

What scientists measure are called variables or factors. They typically distinguish between two kinds of variables: dependent and independent. Dependent variables are the effects of some causes, and in communicative disorders, they are communicative behaviors of all kinds. Normal and disordered speech, language, fluency, and vocal behaviors are all dependent variables. Obviously, these behaviors are a product of known or unknown causal factors. The causal factors of these variables, when experimentally demonstrated, are the independent variables. Simply stated, independent variables are the causes; dependent variables are the effects.

If it is demonstrated, for example, that a child's language behaviors are determined by certain parental reactions, then those specific reactions are the independent variables, and the child's language behaviors are the dependent variables. Similarly, if it is shown that stuttering is due to some genes a person inherits, then those genes are the independent variables, whereas stuttering is the dependent variable.

Scientists start with some effects or dependent variables and proceed to find out their independent variables. The effect may be an eclipse, an earthquake, a chemical reaction, a behavioral problem such as crime, or a disorder of communication. Generally speaking, the same effects may be produced by several causes, and this is the concept of multiple causation. An articulation disorder, for example, may be the result of several factors including low intelligence, an organic defect, poor environmental stimulation, and faulty contingencies of reinforcement. Stuttering may be due to a genetic predisposition combined with situational stress, anxiety, punishment of some aspects of speech, or reinforcement of dysfluencies. Delayed language may result from neural damage, along with a lack of environmental stimulation and parental interactions. It is important to note that these are only potential independent variables; there is no suggestion here that they have been demonstrated to be the causes of those communicative disorders. The examples serve only to show that there may be numerous potential independent variables (causes) for a given dependent variable (effect).

The scientist's task is to isolate a specific cause of a given effect. In order to demonstrate that a certain variable is indeed an independent variable, one will have to rule out all other variables that may also be causes of the effect under investigation. To take a clinical example, if a clinician wishes to establish the effects of a new treatment for language disorders, this treatment must be applied in the absence of all other intervention procedures. While the treatment is applied to a child, for instance, it must be ascertained that the parents at home are not doing something that might stimulate language. Similarly, a teacher might institute a new language program in the classroom that would affect the child's language, and this too must be controlled.

Essentially, scientific methodology makes it possible for scientists to rule out potential independent variables and establish a cause-and-effect relation between two specific events. A treatment technique that is successful in remediating language disorders in the absence of other potential independent variables can be considered the cause of improved language.

EXPERIMENT

The concept of *experiment* captures the essence of scientific methods. An experiment can be defined as a systematic manipulation of an independent variable under controlled conditions in order to produce changes in a dependent variable. It is a strategy to establish cause-and-effect relations in a scientific manner. It is designed to rule out the influence of potential independent variables the experimenter is not interested in. These are called extraneous independent variables. Manipulation of an independent variable and control of the conditions are the two critical aspects of an experiment. In the example just given, the new language treatment (the independent variable) is applied in some quantity, such as twice a week for 30 minutes each time. The duration as well as the frequency of sessions may be increased or decreased, and the amount of reinforcement for correct responses may be higher or lower. Changes such as these constitute manipulation of an independent variable.

The independent variable must be manipulated under controlled conditions. This means the clinician must follow certain procedures to rule out the influence of potential extraneous independent variables, such as the teacher's language stimulation program, or developmental changes over time.

There are two basic strategies to rule out the influence of extraneous independent variables and thereby establish a cause-and-effect relation between any two variables. In clinical situations, the same two strategies are used to establish the effectiveness of treatment programs. These strategies are described in a later section.

SCIENCE AND CLINICAL PRACTICE

Historically, there has been an unfortunate division between clinical practice and scientific research. Several misconceptions seem to underlie this artificial division. It is often thought that scientific research is basic and clinical activity is applied; that scientific research is rigorous, but clinical practice is more or less informal; that scientists find out what the clinicians ought to do, and clinicians then can go ahead and do it; that speech-language pathology is a humanistic and helping profession, while scientific research is cold and mechanical; and that clinicians need not spend much time studying the concepts and methods of science, because clinical practice is inherently different from scientific work. Misconceptions such as these have affected the training of speech-language pathologists, and in turn the nature of clinical practice. Fortunately, in recent years, many clinicians and scientists in the field have questioned these stereotypic notions (Costello, 1979; Minifie, 1983; Ringel, 1972).

Similarities Between Scientific and Clinical Activities

There are some striking similarities between the work of scientists and that of clinicians. The starting point of either scientific or clinical activity is a problem, a question, or a situation that demands analytic attention. Whether the problem or the question is basic or applied, clinical or nonclinical, it requires an answer. The question may concern the movement of stars or the causes and treatment of a speech disorder. At this point, both the scientist and the clinician will have identified a particular phenomenon for investigation. The next step usually involves gathering whatever information is available on that phenomenon. This is the stage of description, and it is common to both scientific and clinical work. A scientist reviews past studies and their results and thus identifies the need for further work. At this stage, the scientist refines the problem in need of investigation.

The first thing the clinician does is determine exactly what problem needs professional help. If the clinician did not know the previously researched information on the disorder, that information is reviewed first. The next step is to make an assessment of the problem by measuring and describing the behaviors the client exhibits (or does not exhibit). Thus, the initial clinical operations such as gathering the client's history and making an assessment are very similar to the scientist's initial work of reviewing the literature and describing the problem to be investigated. In this process, the scientist and the clinician will have specified their dependent variable, which is the effect the scientist wishes to explain, and the disorder the clinician wishes to treat.

Once the phenomenon or a disorder has been clearly identified and described, the scientist proceeds to the actual investigation, and the clinician, to the treatment. In the investigation, the scientist will be most interested in isolating the independent variable of the phenomenon. Typically, the scientist arranges an experimental situation under controlled conditions and then manipulates an independent variable to see if the effect can thus be changed. If it is, the cause of the event will have been isolated.

The clinician, too, needs to identify certain independent variables in order to modify the disorder. The independent variables that are manipulated in treatment situations may or may not be the original causes of the disorder. They may be maintaining factors that, when changed, will change the disorder. In any case, clinical treatment variables applied by the clinician are very similar to the independent variables manipulated by the scientist.

In scientific research, when causes of an event are isolated under controlled conditions, and the same causes have been replicated by other scientists, the event will have been explained. In the majority of scientific disciplines, gaining control over an event is probably the key to an explanation. If the event can be reproduced or changed by the scientist, then it is being controlled. Similarly, in clinical practice, when effectiveness of the same treatment variables is replicated by different clinicians in different clients, then the disorder is being manipulated or controlled. Successful treatment of a disorder can eventually lead to an explanation of that disorder.

When events are successfully controlled and explained, they can also be predicted. This chain of prediction and control is one of the highest goals of scientific activities. Similarly, in clinical practice, successful control (treatment) and prediction (prognosis and prevention) are among the highest of the clinical goals.

An Important Distinction

At least one important difference between routine clinical work and scientific research must be recognized, however. The difference lies in the amount of care taken to rule out the influence of extraneous independent variables. In scientific research, a great deal of care is taken to make sure that the only independent variable active in an experiment is the one the scientist is interested in. Steps are taken to rule out the influence of potential causes that are extraneous to the purposes of the study. This is rarely done in routine clinical work. If it has been demonstrated that a given treatment procedure is effective, the clinician simply uses it. Typically, not much is done to make sure that the client is not simultaneously exposed to other formal or informal treatment procedures. To the extent that extraneous treatments are considered helpful, such an exposure may be even promoted by the clinician.

The distinction is valid only when routine clinical work is compared with controlled laboratory research. The distinction is not as clear when clinical research is compared with basic or nonclinical research. In fact, there are no significant procedural differences between controlled clinical and laboratory research. Both kinds of research seek to isolate a cause-and-effect relation between two events. The clinical researcher may wish to isolate the original or the maintaining cause of a given disorder, or an effective treatment for it. In achieving these goals, however, the clinical researcher must follow the same procedures the scientist follows. Just like the scientist, the clinical researcher rules out extraneous independent variables, manipulates a specific independent variable (treatment), produces changes in a dependent variable (communicative behavior or disorder), and thus establishes a cause-and-effect relation between the treatment and client behavior.

IMPROVEMENT VERSUS EFFECTIVENESS

The fact that in routine clinical work nothing is done to rule out the influence of other potential treatment variables leads to an important distinction between improvement in client behaviors and effectiveness of treatment techniques.

Typically, the clinician will have assessed the client's communicative behaviors to determine the need for clinical services. Thus, the fact that the client lacks certain speech, language, voice, or fluency behaviors will have been documented. Baselines of target behaviors will strengthen these assessment data. Typically, treatment follows. After a period of time, the client may begin to produce the target behaviors that he or she did not produce before the treatment. Throughout the treatment period, the clinician measures the target behaviors to show systematic changes in those behaviors under treatment. Before the treatment is terminated, an additional measure is taken to show that the client has learned what was taught during the treatment sessions. With this, the clinician usually concludes that the client has improved with the help of clinical services. As long as changes in client behaviors were documented, the claim regarding improvement may be acceptable. Such documented changes also demonstrate clinician accountability.

The fact that the client improved while receiving treatment does not necessarily suggest that the treatment was indeed effective, however. Improvement is a necessary but not a sufficient condition for establishing effectiveness of treatment techniques. In uncontrolled treatment, there is no assurance that clients could not have produced those behaviors in the absence of treatment. In other words, what are considered "normal developmental changes" are not ruled out by clinicians. Similarly, the potential influence of formal or informal treatment programs initiated by people other than the clinician is not ruled out. As a result, clinicians normally cannot claim effectiveness for treatment programs used in routine clinical work.

Clinician accountability, therefore, means that the changes in the client behaviors were objectively demonstrated. In routine clinical situations, clinicians are not able to demonstrate effectiveness of treatment procedures, partly because the traditional techniques of establishing treatment effectiveness are cumbersome, impractical, and difficult to use with clients. An alternative approach, which offers more practical methods of evaluating treatment techniques, is available. Both of these approaches are described in the next section.

The distinction between client improvement and treatment effectiveness highlights the importance of controlled clinical research. Treatment techniques can be advocated only on the basis of controlled evidence. Unfortunately, many "treatment procedures" are often recommended in the absence of such evidence. In due course some of those procedures begin to be used in routine clinical work without ever having been evaluated experimentally.

DOCUMENTING TREATMENT EFFECTIVENESS

As was indicated before, legal, social, scientific, and professional considerations point up the need for more careful documentation of the effects of treatment techniques used by speech-language pathologists. It is often thought that clinical researchers will establish the effectiveness of treatment by following the methods of science, and that routine clinical work need not be burdened by such a requirement. While it is quite possible that a majority of clinical activity will always remain uncontrolled, this idea has been taken to such extremes in our profession that it has hurt us professionally.

All clinicians must thoroughly understand the basic set of procedures by which systematic observations are made, measurements are taken, and cause-and-effect relations are established. Demonstrating treatment effectiveness is a matter of establishing a cause-and-effect relation between certain procedures implemented by the clinician and changes in client behaviors. Technically speaking, treatment effects are not demonstrated until such a cause-and-effect relation is established. Even if most clinicians are not going to do research, they are still expected to be consumers of scientific information. Unless clinicians have a good grasp of the methods of science and experimentation, it is doubtful whether they can be informed consumers of technical information. The only sure consequence of a lack of knowledge of science and its methods is that the clinician will continuously lag behind developments in the profession.

Clinicians ought to be critical consumers of research. It is not enough to merely understand research studies; the results of studies must be evaluated. Unless clinicians understand the concepts and methods of science, they may not be able to evaluate research information. Critical evaluation is especially important in the realm of treatment techniques. The clinician must be able to judge whether the new or the old treatment procedures have been tested out in actual clinical practice, and, if so, what kind of evidence is available regarding their effectiveness. An unfortunate consequence of not being a critical consumer is that the clinician is endlessly swayed by faddish developments in the profession. Every profession has its share of such developments, which may be perceived as revolutions and breakthroughs. A critical clinician is able to distinguish those treatment procedures whose effects are experimentally demonstrated from those that are based on logic, rational arguments, and uncontrolled clinical applications.

It is also possible that a better understanding of experimental procedures will encourage more clinicians to gather controlled evidence that might be supportive of clinical practices. Such evidence can be expected to help improve treatment procedures as well.

In the following sections, we will describe two basic approaches to documenting effectiveness of treatment programs: the between-groups strategy and the within-subject strategy.

THE BETWEEN-GROUPS STRATEGY

The first, and traditional, method of documenting treatment effectiveness is based on the concept of group comparisons. It is variously known by such names as between-groups strategy, group design method, or statistical research designs. The basic idea in this approach is that clients who are treated will change while those who are not treated remain unchanged. The method requires two groups of subjects who are comparable in terms of age, intelligence, family and social background, educational level, the type and severity of the disorder being treated, and other such characteristics. One group is the experimental group, which receives treatment; the other is the control group, which does not.

With the group comparison method, it is very important to make sure that the subjects in the two groups are indeed similar on all of the relevant variables. Such a similarity can be achieved either by the random procedure or by matching.

The Random Procedure

This is based on the statistical theory of probability. If one selects a certain number of persons from a very large group of people without any bias whatsoever, then those few persons will be representative of the larger group. The larger reference group is called a population, and the selected smaller group is called a sample. A population is any defined group that includes all of the members that possess certain characteristics. All language handicapped children in public schools, and all hearing impaired adults in the United States, are technically defined as populations. Since it is impractical to observe all persons belonging to a population, we select certain individuals and study them. However, in order to be useful, the results of the study must be relevant to the population, not just to the selected sample. Therefore, special care must be taken to make sure that the sample is representative of the population.

The representativeness of a sample is assured when every subject in the population has had an equal chance of being selected into the study. That is, experimenter bias cannot influence the subject selection process. To achieve this, the subjects are selected on a random basis. Each individual in the population, for example, may be assigned a number, and all odd-numbered persons may be selected for the study. Such random procedures result in samples that represent the population.

The random approach requires that a large population of subjects be available so that a sample can be drawn from it. For clinical research, patients or clients with specific disorders must be available in large numbers. For example, in establishing the effects of a new treatment program for school-age language disordered children, the clinician must have access to a large group of children with that disorder, all of whom are willing to participate in the study. The needed number of children can then be selected on a random basis.

Once the needed numbers of subjects are selected randomly, they are then randomly assigned to the experimental or the control group. That is, experimenter bias should not be a factor in deciding who gets treated and who does not. Random assignment of subjects to the experimental and control groups creates two comparable groups. Thus, the random procedure must be used at two levels: first in selecting the subjects from the larger population, and then in assigning them to either the experimental or the control group. When this is done, the clinician can assume that the subjects in the two groups are similar with regard to the relevant variables, such as socioeconomic status, intelligence, family background, and the type and severity of the disorder to be treated.

Matching

An alternative to random procedure is matching. This procedure is also designed to give the clinical researcher two comparable groups. In matching, the clinician makes sure that the specific types of subjects included in the two groups are similar. Matched groups need not necessarily represent the population, but they are comparable to each other. For example, if the experimental group consisted of 15 five year old language disordered children with average intelligence, coming from middle-class families, and living in suburbs, the control group should also consist of 15 children with the same characteristics.

When certain disorders are the dependent variables, as they are in most clinical research, the duration, the specific types, and the severity of the disorder should all be factors considered in matching subjects. For example, in a study involving articulation disorders, if the subjects in the experimental group are considered to have "functional" articulation disorder, those in the control group cannot have "neurologically based" articulation disorder. When the experimental group subjects have been stuttering for five years, the control group subjects should also have been stuttering for five years. If the children in one of the language disordered groups are nonverbal, those in the other group should also be nonverbal.

Experimentation

The formation of two groups, either randomized or matched, sets the stage for the actual experimentation. Before the treatment is started, the relevant behaviors such as language, stuttering, or articulation are measured. These measures are known as pretests. The treatment technique whose effects must be established is then applied to subjects in the experimental group. The control group subjects go without treatment until the experiment is over. After the experimental group has received treatment for a duration considered appropriate, the communicative behaviors of subjects in both the groups are again evaluated. This second evaluation is known as the posttest.

The effects of the treatment procedure are determined by a comparison of the two posttest measures. If the treatment was effective, the two posttest measures will be significantly different from each other. For the most part, results generated by group experimental designs are analyzed by statistical procedures such as analysis of variance or t tests. When the groups are comparable to begin with, significant difference on the posttest must be attributed to the treatment itself. In such cases, it is assumed that none of the potential extraneous independent variables were responsible for the significant changes observed in the experimental group, because if they were, the members of the control group would also have shown similar changes. Of course, should the subjects in the control group also show changes in their communicative behaviors, the effects of the treatment procedure would remain questionable.

The experimental group-control group design just described is one of the basic group designs. There are several different designs within this strategy, and each design also has its variations. It is not the purpose of this chapter to review clinical research designs. Rather, it is to give some basic information on the need to establish treatment effectiveness in order to point out the importance of studying research methods in some detail.

Limitations of the Between-Groups Strategy

Because of some basic requirements of the between-groups strategy, it is especially difficult to use in clinical sciences. First, it is not easy to find a large number of persons (population) with a given disorder who are accessible and willing to participate in the study. It is difficult to gain access to populations of language disordered children, stutterers, aphasic persons, those with laryngectomies, or the hearing impaired. As a result, clinical research is often done with subjects who happen to seek professional services, which means that the subjects are not randomly selected from their respective populations. The fact that the available subjects are randomly assigned to either the experimental or the control group will not assure the representativeness of the sample.

Second, the matching procedure is also very difficult to implement. It may not be possible to find subjects with specific clinical disorders of the same type and severity that also have the same personal, social, family, and educational characteristics. Consequently, very few experimental clinical studies are done with matched subjects.

Third, the requirement of a control group that does not receive treatment may pose some practical and ethical problems. If the clients can be given the needed help, it may be undesirable to deny or postpone treatment for the sake of research. In some clinical research, patients on the waiting list have served as the control group, but this presumes the existence of a large number of patients waiting for services. Many researchers in communicative disorders cannot realize this situation. Even if they do, the waiting list–based control group would not be a matched or randomly selected sample.

Fourth, enough clients to form two groups of subjects just may not be available, irrespective of the random procedure. The clinical researcher might wait forever looking for 30 or 40 dysarthric persons who share similar personal, social, and other characteristics, all of whom are simultaneously available for research.

Fifth, group designs are not conducive to intensive observation of individual subjects, which is often needed in clinical sciences. Results obtained from larger samples are usually analyzed in terms of the statistical mean. Such average performances do not give a clear picture of individual performances and differences. On the basis of such studies, it is difficult for the clinician to determine whether a given client will also benefit from the researched procedure.

Sixth, the between-groups methodology does not give a total perspective of changes in client behaviors across treatment sessions. Since normally only two measures are obtained (once before and once after the treatment), it is not possible to see change in real time. With this method, the clinician is not able to monitor the techniques or modify them during treatment sessions.

For these reasons, we do not find many experimental studies in clinical fields that use the group methodology in an appropriate manner. Studies that do use this approach often sacrifice the random procedure by selecting subjects who are available for research. As such, the most critical aspect of the group methodology is omitted in practice.

THE WITHIN-SUBJECT STRATEGY

An alternative to the group strategy is available and is being used in many clinical sciences. The approach, known as the within-subject or single-subject strategy, was developed in the intensive study of individual subjects. The goal of the single-subject strategy is to isolate cause-and-effect relations among behavioral events. Typically, a specified independent variable is systematically manipulated to see if the dependent variables (behaviors) show corresponding changes. The methodology is especially suited to clinical sciences that study individual clients intensively.

Within the single-subject approach, many subjects are not observed just once or twice, which is more frequently done in the group strategy. Instead, fewer individuals are repeatedly observed. Since clinicians tend to see the same few clients over and over again, this methodology has been found to be very suitable to answering clinical research questions. Additionally, this approach is not based on the random procedure, and therefore, there is no need to have an access to a large clinical population that is willing to participate in the study.

Most of the single-subject designs do not require matching, since the approach is not based on group comparisons. Normally, there is no control group that does not receive treatment. As a result, the problems associated with not treating a control group are avoided. Instead, each subject serves as his or her own control. The clients receive treatment in one condition, and do not receive treatment in another condition. The same client's behaviors under treatment versus no treatment are compared to determine the effects of treatment. Since there is no need to compare one subject's performance with that of another subject, each individual is treated as unique in the single subject methodology.

Another characteristic of the single-subject methodology is that the subjects' behaviors are measured continuously. Treatment effects are not determined on the basis of pretest and posttest measures only. The behaviors for which the treatment is applied are measured in each experimental session so that a continuous picture of change over time is obtained.

There are several single-subject designs to determine treatment effectiveness, and it is not possible to review all of them. We shall take a look at the following three single-subject designs: the ABA, the ABAB, and the multiple baseline design. These are the most frequently used single-subject designs in documenting treatment effectiveness, although ABA is not a clinical design.

A common feature of most single-subject designs is the establishment of baselines before the application of treatment. Baselines refer to pretreatment measures of behaviors. The methodology requires that the baseline be reliable. Therefore, within single-subject designs, the behaviors are measured repeatedly to establish a stable trend in the frequency of those behaviors.

As an example, suppose a clinician wishes to find out if a certain training program will be effective in teaching certain morphologic features to language delayed children. The first thing to do is to establish the frequency with which the children are using the selected features. The children may not be producing the features at all (zero frequency), or they may be producing them at some low frequency. The exact frequency of the selected morphologic features (between 0 and 100 percent) must be measured through language samples or other means. To establish reliability, two or more samples must be obtained. A stable baserate is considered to have been established when multiple measures are consistent with each other. If the measures differ widely, then the language sampling is continued until the frequency of morphologic use across two or three samples is stable. Detailed procedures of establishing baselines of communicative behaviors are described in Chapter 5.

After the baselines of target behaviors have been established, the treatment is initiated. The phases subsequent to treatment can be somewhat different across designs, and for this reason, the designs will be described separately.

The ABA Design

The ABA is one of the original experimental designs developed in the study of single subjects. In the initial A phase, the baselines are established. In the next B phase, the treatment is applied. The treatment is continued until changes in the target behaviors are unquestionable. Then in the final A phase, the treatment is withdrawn.

The logic of the design is simple. If the behaviors were stable during the baserate condition (A), but changed during the treatment (B), and returned to the baserate when the treatment was withdrawn (second A), then the treatment was probably the single effective agent. If extraneous variables were active, then the changes would have continued even after the treatment was withdrawn.

Obviously, the design should not be used if the objective is to have the treatment effects last. This is why it was said earlier that the ABA is not a *clinical* design. Nevertheless, it can establish the effects of an independent variable or a treatment program in an unambiguous manner. A variation of this basic ABA design can fulfill the clinical requirements in that the design ends with an extended period of treatment. This is the ABAB design to be described next.

The ABAB Design

The ABAB design has two versions: withdrawal and reversal. The first three conditions of the ABAB withdrawal are identical with the basic ABA design just described. First, the target behaviors are baserated. Second, the treatment is applied to those behaviors. Third, the treatment is withdrawn, as in the ABA design. These three conditions of the design will demonstrate the experimental control over the target behaviors if the selected treatment was an effective variable. However, after having demonstrated the declining trend in the behaviors when the treatment was withdrawn, the clinician reapplies the treatment in the final B phase of the design. The treatment is typically continued as long as it takes to achieve the goal of intervention. Thus, in the ABAB withdrawal design, the treatment is withdrawn once, and applied twice, to show that the behaviors changed when the treatment was initially applied, changed again when it was withdrawn, and changed a third time when it was reapplied.

The ABAB reversal design is identical with the ABAB withdrawal design in terms of all but the second A phase. After the initial baselines are established, the treatment is first applied to the target behaviors; then, the treatment is not simply withdrawn but is applied to the incompatible or error responses briefly. This is done to demonstrate that when the treatment was applied to the error responses, they increased in frequency while the target behaviors showed a simultaneous decrease. In the treatment of an articulation disorder, for example, the correct production of the selected target phoneme may be baserated initially and reinforced in the first B phase. In the second A phase, the incorrect productions may be reinforced for a brief time to see whether the correct production decreases and the incorrect production increases. If such results are seen, the experimental control of the reinforcement contingency will have been demonstrated.

In the final phase of the ABAB reversal design, the target behaviors are once again treated. The treatment is continued until the final goals of the program are achieved.

Figure 2–1, reproduced from a language training study (Hegde and McConn, 1981) illustrates the ABAB reversal design. In this study, "probes" were conducted between experimental phases to assess generalization of treatment effects. The probe procedures are described in Chapter 5. Note that although the trained production (auxiliary *are*) was reversed briefly, the study was terminated only when the target feature was produced and generalized at a high level.

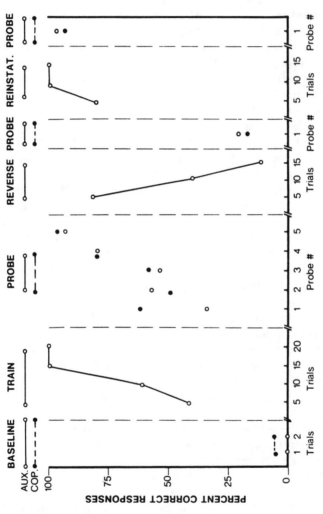

Figure 2–1.   Percent correct responses of auxiliary and copula are across the experimental conditions when only the auxiliary was trained, reversed, and reinstated in a 22 year old female subject. The graph shows the baseline, experimental, probe, reversal, and reinstatement conditions of an ABAB design. From Hegde, M. N., and McConn, J. (1981). Language Training: Some data on response classes and generalization to an occupational setting. *Journal of Speech and Hearing Disorders, 46,* 353–358. Reprinted with permission.

Incidentally, the graph also shows that the experimental manipulations of auxiliary had corresponding effects on copula as well.

Both versions of the ABAB design rule out the influence of extraneous independent variables, including maturational factors. If some extraneous variables were to be responsible for the treatment effect, then the target behaviors would not decrease when the treatment is either withdrawn or reversed.

One of the problems with the ABAB design is that in order to rule out the extraneous independent variables, the treatment effect is neutralized (withdrawal) or reversed (incorrect responses reinforced). Though this is done for a very brief period of time, it can still be somewhat inefficient from the standpoint of clinical intervention. In some cases, it may be totally undesirable to withdraw or reverse treatment. In certain clients, it may be difficult to reduce or eliminate a trained behavior for short times. In such cases, reversal training may have to be extensive, which is obviously undesirable. Normally, behaviors are reversed during early stages of training when they are not yet firmly established, but the difficulty in reversing a target behavior can still be faced.

A design that avoids the problems of the ABAB designs is available. It permits conclusions about the effectiveness of treatment without reversal or withdrawal of treatment. It is called the multiple baseline design, and in several respects, it is one of the best of the clinical designs.

The Multiple Baseline Design

The multiple baseline design has three variations: multiple baseline across behaviors, across settings, and across subjects. The multiple baselines refer to either several target behaviors, treatment settings, or clients.

In routine clinical situations, the multiple baseline design across behaviors is probably easier to implement than the other two variations. The design requires that at least three target behaviors be treated in a given client. This poses no problem to the clinician because most clients need to acquire more than one target behavior anyway. This is especially true of clients with language and articulation disorders.

In using the multiple baseline design, the clinician first establishes baselines on all of the selected target behaviors. If a child with an articulation disorder were to receive treatment on four phonemes, these are baserated with a certain number of words each. Then the treatment is started on the first phoneme. The phoneme may be trained at the word level to a specified performance criterion. As soon as the child reaches this criterion, the clinician would normally move to the next phoneme. Within the multiple baseline design, instead of starting the treatment right away on a different phoneme, the baselines of the remaining three untrained phonemes are repeated. If the treatment were the only factor involved, the percent correct production of the three untrained phonemes would not show significant change from the initial baseline.

The next step is to train the second phoneme to the performance criterion. As soon as this is accomplished, the baselines of the remaining two untrained phonemes are reestablished. Once again, these baselines are expected to be comparable with the first two baselines. The third phoneme is then trained, followed by another baseline of the last phoneme, which is then trained to the criterion. In this manner, baseline and training are alternated until all of the target behaviors are trained.

Figure 2–2, reproduced from a language training study (Hegde and Gierut, 1979) illustrates the multiple baselines across behaviors. Note that four grammatical features were sequentially trained in the same subjects. Each subsequent behavior had more baseline trials, and none of the behaviors under baseline changed.

In the design involving multiple baselines across settings, the same behavior of the same client is baserated and sequentially trained in different settings. For example, production of selected manual signs by a hard of hearing child may be baserated in the clinic, in the regular classroom, and in the special classroom the child attends for a few hours each day. Assuming that the target signs are not produced in any of these settings, the training is started in one of the settings. After the behaviors reach the training criterion in that setting, the sign productions are baserated a second time in the remaining two "untrained" settings. The training is then started in the second setting, followed by the last baseline in the third setting. Finally, the training is started in the third setting. If the signs are produced only in the setting where they were trained, but absent in settings not involved in training, then the clinician will have demonstrated experimental control.

The multiple baseline across subjects involves the same behavior in different subjects. Reduction of hypernasal speech production, for example, may be the treatment target in four children with repaired cleft. The production of nonnasal speech sounds with nasal resonance is initially baserated across these children. One of the children is then trained to the training criterion in the nonnasal production of target speech sounds in words. The target behavior in the other three subjects is baserated a second time, followed by training of the second

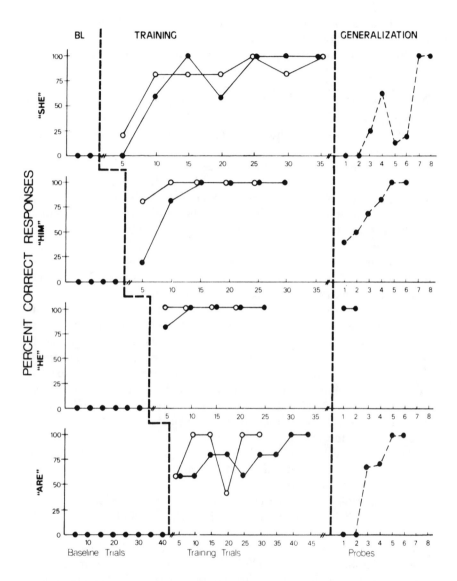

Figure 2–2. Percent correct verbal responses on baseline, training, and probe trials for the four behaviors trained in a language delayed child (4.9 years). The training segments of the graph represent responses given to two training items in the case of each behavior. The graph illustrates the use of the multiple baseline design across behaviors. From Hegde, M. N., and Gierut, J. (1979). The operant training and generalization of pronouns and a verb form in a language delayed child. *Journal of Communication Disorders, 12,* 23–34. Reprinted with permission.

child. In this manner, training and baselines are alternated across children until all of them are trained.

It must be noted that multiple baseline design across subjects comes very close to the traditional matched-subjects design. Subjects who do not receive treatment serve the control function the way they do in many group designs. Therefore, the selected subjects should be comparable in their relevant characteristics. For this reason, the design shares some of the problems associated with the matched-group design.

With the multiple baseline design, the clinician hopes to show that the frequency of a given target behavior increased only when it came under the clinician's training procedure. In the across-behaviors version, the frequency of behaviors of the same client should remain unchanged until they are picked up for training by the clinician. In the across-settings version, the trained behavior should not be produced in untreated settings. In the across-subjects version, the untreated subjects should not show changes in the target behaviors. In this manner, potential extraneous variables are ruled out.

An attractive feature of the design is that it can be used in routine clinical work. It does not alter clinical service in any significant manner. The necessary components of the design are a part of responsible clinical work. For example, the design requires that the target behaviors be baserated. This is a normal clinical procedure used to document the need for clinical services. The repeated baselines are also necessary from the standpoint of everyday clinical practice, since a baseline established earlier must be repeated immediately before the training is initiated on that behavior.

There are other single-subject strategies, such as the alternating treatment design and interactional design. In the former, the relative effects of two or more treatments can be assessed, whereas in the latter, independent and interactive effects of more than one treatment can be established. Interested clinicians should refer to some of the several excellent sources on single subject designs (Barlow, Hayes, and Nelson, 1984; Barlow and Hersen, 1984; McReynolds and Kearns, 1983). In addition, clinical studies published in professional journals can be helpful in understanding these and other methods of establishing treatment effectiveness. Throughout this book, clinical studies documenting treatment effectiveness are cited.

GENERALITY OF TREATMENT EFFECTS

Generally speaking, the effectiveness of treatment programs is initially demonstrated by one or a few researchers using a certain number of clients. Either the between-groups or the within-subjects strategy may be used for this purpose. Once this is done, the next scientific task is to show that the technique can be effective with other clients, when used by other clinicians, and in other professional settings. When this task is accomplished to a certain extent, the technique is considered to have some generality.

The basic method in establishing the generality of treatment effects is to replicate the research studies in different settings. This is typically done by other clinicians involving clients who are similar to those in the original study. Replications may also include clients who in some respects differ from those in the original study. For example, if the original study had demonstrated effectiveness of a language training procedure with five year old children, a replicated study can be made to find out if similar results can be achieved with older or younger children, or even with adult clients.

The importance of the issue of generality of treatment effects cannot be overemphasized. Unless it is known that different clinicians have obtained favorable results in different professional settings (clinics, hospitals, public school settings) a technique may not be recommended for general use. An initial failure to establish generality of a technique does not always suggest that it is ineffective. It is possible that those who tried to replicate the study did not apply the technique correctly. When this is not the case, lack of generality limits the usefulness of the technique. Even then, it may be found that the technique works well with specific types of clients or disorders.

SELECTION OF TREATMENT PROCEDURES

A problem clinicians often face is the selection of treatment procedures. Even an informal review of treatment literature in communicative disorders reveals a variety of descriptions of how to remediate specific disorders. Some of the standard controversies in the field are concerned with how to train clients with language and articulation disorders, stuttering, or hearing impairment. Sometimes clinicians may find it difficult to select treatment procedures because contradictory approaches may be equally appealing, especially when each is considered alone. This is particularly true when different procedures are described in a logically consistent manner. In other words, the descriptions of procedures may have logical validity. The descriptions may also be scholarly and therefore impressive. Nevertheless, when there are alternative treatment procedures, the clinician has to select.

In some cases, subjective factors may influence the selection of treatment techniques. The clinician may know and like the author or may be impressed with the descriptions of the technique. The clinician may think that it is easy to use the technique, or may find it inherently appealing. The author may be well known and considered an authority on the subject. Obviously, factors such as these are irrelevant to the treatment selection process.

Probably the single most important criterion of treatment selection is the presence or absence of controlled and replicated evidence. The technique must have been experimentally evaluated to show that it can be effective in the absence of other potential treatment procedures. It must have been used by different clinicians in different settings with similar results. The (presumed) effectiveness of the technique should not depend upon such vague factors as the "personality" of the clinician or the clinician-client "chemistry," or "good rapport." These factors are often lame excuses for ineffective techniques.

In selecting treatment procedure, then, the clinician should ask three basic questions. (1) Has the technique been experimentally evaluated? (2) Have the results been favorable? (3) Has the technique been replicated across settings, clinicians, and clients? If the answer is positive to all three questions, the clinician is justified in using the technique in routine clinical situations.

Unfortunately, answers to these questions are not always clear. Different viewpoints may be supported to different degrees. However, evidence in favor of a variety of techniques can often be found on a hierarchy. Some techniques are based purely on speculative but logically consistent and scholarly reasoning. These are the most suspect of the techniques. Some techniques are based on uncontrolled case studies. There are data to show that when such a technique is used systematically, the clients improve, but there is no assurance that in the absence of other potential treatment techniques, it can still produce favorable results. Such techniques may be used on a tentative basis. At the next level, the clinician may find treatment procedures that have been experimentally evaluated and are found to be effective. There may not be replicated evidence, however. The clinician can use these techniques with a certain degree of confidence while being watchful of possible replications. The most desirable techniques are those that present favorable, controlled, and replicated evidence with known limits of generality.

The emphasis placed upon the use of experimentally evaluated techniques is not meant to discourage creative clinical work. The clinicians should always be willing to try new techniques. While doing this, however, the clinician should be fully aware that something unproved is being tried. The clinician must be scrupulously careful in measuring client behaviors, keeping objective records, and systematically (even if informally) evaluating the technique in the context of each client. In this context, the clinician who can use some of the single-subject designs can produce controlled evidence in favor of the technique being used while providing clinical services. Techniques such as multiple baseline designs can be very useful in this regard.

SUMMARY

There is a growing recognition in the profession of communicative disorders of the need to strengthen the scientific bases of our profession.

Speech-language pathologists must adopt the philosophy of science, learn dispositions of science, and apply the methods of science to the study of the subject matter. The most critical aspect of science that needs to be used more often is the method of experimentation.

Scientific and clinical work share several common characteristics. Both science and clinical work seek to analyze phenomena, determine cause-and-effect relations between events, modify the effects of certain variables, and predict and control events. Unlike science, most clinical activity is uncontrolled, however.

"Client improvement" refers to changes in behaviors under treatment. Treatment effectiveness, which is not the same as improvement, is documented only when the influence of other potential treatment variables is ruled out.

Clinicians should understand the philosophy, methodology, and dispositions of science so that they can be critical consumers of technical information. They must know the methods by which treatment effects are established.

There are two methods of establishing treatment effectiveness: the between-groups strategy and the within-subject strategy. The former approach is based on the statistical theories of probability, random samples, and group performance differences, which are evaluated statistically. The latter approach is based on intensive study of individual clients. Each has its strengths and weaknesses. By and large, the within-subject strategy is more suitable for clinical research.

Replication is the method by which the generality of treatment effects is demonstrated. Eventually, generality across settings, clinicians, and clients must be established for each treatment technique.

The degree to which a treatment technique is based upon controlled evidence, replicated evidence, or both should determine its selection or rejection.

STUDY GUIDE

Answer the following questions in technical language. Check your answers with the text. Rewrite your answers when necessary.

1. Define science.
2. What are some of the popular misconceptions of science?
3. What are some of the assumptions of science as a philosophy?
4. What is the meaning of objective procedures?
5. Define dependent variables.
6. Define independent variables.
7. Are communicative disorders typically dependent or independent variables?
8. What kinds of variables are treatment techniques?
9. Give at least two specific examples each of independent and dependent variables.
10. What is an experiment?
11. What is meant by "manipulations of an independent variable"?
12. Define control.
13. What are extraneous independent variables?
14. Describe the similarities between scientific and clinical activity.
15. Compare and contrast scientific experiment and clinical treatment.
16. When is an event "explained"?
17. What are among the highest scientific as well as clinical goals?
18. What is an important distinction between scientific research and routine clinical work?
19. Are there critical distinctions between clinical research and non-clinical research?
20. Distinguish between improvement and effectiveness.
21. State the reasons why a clinician cannot necessarily claim effectiveness even though the client improved under treatment.
22. Specify why the clinician who does not wish to do research should still understand the methods of science by which treatment effects are established.
23. Who is a critical consumer of research information?
24. Describe between-subjects strategy.
25. Define within-subject strategy.
26. What is a random procedure?
27. Define population and sample.
28. Distinguish between random selection and random assignment.
29. What is matching?
30. Distinguish between experimental group and control group.

31. How are the results of the group experimental designs analyzed?
32. State the limitations of the between-groups strategy.
33. What are the general characteristics of the within-subject strategy?
34. What is an ABAB design?
35. Describe the reversal design.
36. Define a withdrawal design.
37. What are the limitations of the ABA and ABAB designs?
38. What is a multiple baseline design?
39. What are the variations of a multiple baseline design?
40. What are the problems with the multiple baseline design across subjects?
41. Why are single-subject designs more applicable to clinical research?
42. Define generality.
43. What are the three major kinds of generalities?
44. What are some of the subjective factors that might influence the treatment selection process?
45. What are the specified objective criteria for the selection of treatment techniques?
46. Describe the hierarchical arrangement of clinical evidence.
47. How should a clinician use treatment techniques that have not been verified?
48. What kind of knowledge or expertise will help in the process of evaluating treatment effectiveness?

REFERENCES

Bachrach, A. J. (1969). *Psychological research: An introduction.* New York: Random House.

Barlow, D. H., Hayes, S. C., and Nelson, R. O. (1984). *The scientist practitioner.* New York: Pergamon.

Barlow, D. H., and Hersen, M. (1984). *Single case experimental designs: Strategies for studying behavior change.* New York: Pergamon.

Costello, J. M. (1979). Clinicians and researchers: A necessary dichotomy? *Journal of National Student Speech and Hearing Association, 7,* 6–26.

Hegde, M. N., and Gierut, J. (1979). The operant training and generalization of pronouns and a verb form in a language delayed child. *Journal of Communication Disorders, 12,* 23–34.

Hegde, M. N., and McConn, J. (1981). Language training: Some data on response classes and generalization to an occupational setting. *Journal of Speech and Hearing Disorders, 46,* 353–358.

Minifie, F. (1983). Knowledge and service: Does the foundation of the profession need shoring up? *Asha, 4,* 29–32

McReynolds, L. V., and Kearns, K. P. (1983). *Single-subject experimental designs in communicative disorders*. Baltimore: University Park Press.

Ringel, R. L. (1972). The clinician and the researcher: An artificial dichotomy. *Asha, 14,* 351–353.

Ringel, R. L., Trachtman, L. E., and Prutting, C. A. (1984). The science in human communication sciences. *Asha, 26,* 33–37.

Skinner, B. F. (1953). *Science and human behavior*. New York: Macmillan.

Zimmermann, G. N. (1984). Knowledge and service: Does the foundation of our science need shoring up? *Asha, 26,* 31–34.

Chapter 3

Selection and Definition of Target Behaviors

In Chapters 1 and 2, a treatment paradigm for communicative disorders and procedures for documenting treatment effectiveness were described.

In Chapter 3, the following points will be described:
- Assessment considerations
- Issues concerning selection and definition of target behaviors
- Criteria of measurement
- The normative and the client-specific strategy for selecting target behaviors
- Response classes
- Constituent and operational definitions

The importance of careful selection of behaviors to be trained cannot be overemphasized. The kinds of behaviors that are selected for training may have an impact on the duration of training, whether trained behaviors will generalize to the clients' everyday situations, whether generalized responses will be maintained over time, and whether the training can be considered successful by clients or parents who seek help. In case of language and articulation disorders, the issue of what to train has been as controversial as the treatment techniques themselves. Recent research on stuttering has indicated that one of the most critical factors in therapeutic success is the type of target behavior selected for treatment (Hegde, 1985). For reasons such as these, some of the major questions and answers regarding how to select behaviors for training will be considered.

Once a behavior is selected for training, how it is defined can make a difference in terms of establishing clinician accountability. In this regard, certain ways of defining target behaviors are more useful than others. Therefore, we shall examine the issue of defining target behaviors.

Before target behaviors are selected and defined, a client's communicative behaviors must be assessed. It is therefore necessary to take an overview of the assessment strategies and associated philosophies.

AN OVERVIEW OF ASSESSMENT STRATEGIES

Assessment (sometimes referred to as diagnostics) of a client's communicative behaviors is the initial step in providing clinical services. As soon as a request or referral is made for professional help, most speech and hearing centers send out a case history form that the clients or parents of young clients fill out and return to the center. Soon thereafter, an appointment is made for an assessment.

The assessment typically begins with an interview in which additional information on the client's problem is obtained. Information supplied by the client or parent on the case history form often needs to be clarified, and the interview usually serves this purpose. Generally speaking, the background information obtained through the interview and the case history covers such areas as the client's birth and developmental history; health, medical, and educational information; family history; specifics on speech and language development; the onset and the course of the disorder; information on prior assessment, treatment, and their results; and occupational and marital information if relevant. The focus of the interview depends on the specific disorder, the age of the client, additional medical or behavioral problems the client may have, and so on. It is not the purpose of this chapter to give detailed information on assessment areas and procedures. The clinician should consult some of the many sources available on the assessment of communicative disorders (Darley and Spriestersbach, 1978; Peterson and Marquardt, 1981).

The actual assessment procedure depends to some extent on the specific information obtained through the case history and interview. An oral-peripheral examination is done to evaluate the integrity of the oral structures. If structural deviations such as cleft palate are noticed, the client is referred to a medical specialist.

During the initial few minutes, informal observations of client behaviors are made so that the clinician can determine what kinds of assessment procedures should be selected. Whether and what types of standardized tests are useful, and what kinds of client-specific procedures may be needed, can be determined during this observation.

For example, if the child is hardly able to produce single words, there is no use selecting an advanced syntactic test for administration.

In a typical assessment procedure, the client's language sample is recorded, and selected standardized tests are administered. Because of certain limitations of standardized tests, it is desirable to use additional procedures. We shall shortly address some of the limitations of standardized tests and suggest alternatives.

Language samples are probably more useful than standardized tests because they are more naturalistic, and the number of opportunities to produce given aspects of language can be increased to the extent necessary. The procedure can involve conversational speech, and for this reason may reflect the natural communicative behaviors of the client with relative accuracy. If the client is a young child, the clinician usually arranges a controlled situation in which pictures, toys, and other stimuli are systematically manipulated to evoke specific responses. With adult clients, the more typical conversational speech can serve the purpose.

Taking an adequate language sample from a young child requires some planning and skill on the part of the clinician. Selected stimulus materials must be controlled by the clinician, not by the child. Often, toys and objects more readily evoke play activity than verbal responses. Therefore, the selected stimulus materials must be controlled in order to evoke speech, not to keep the child happy during the assessment.

While evoking speech from the child, the clinician should not talk too much. When too much time is spent talking to the child, he or she may not have enough opportunities to speak. The clinician's speech should serve as verbal cues for speech from the child. For this reason, it is not useful to ask questions that can be answered "yes" or "no." Yes-no questions tend to evoke nonverbal behaviors (such as nodding or shaking the head) from many children. Questions must be open-ended. For example, questions and requests like "what is this?" or "tell me about this picture" or "what did you do yesterday?" may be more effective than "is this a car?" or "is the cat jumping?" or "do you like it?"

The extent to which the clinician must manipulate the stimulus material in a language sampling procedure depends upon the verbal level of the child and the complexity of the language structures to be evoked. If the client is fairly verbal, not much concrete stimulus manipulation may be needed. The child may then be engaged in conversational speech. Generally speaking, the less verbal the child, the greater the need for stimulus manipulation by the clinician. In addition, the more complex the structure to be evoked, the greater the extent of stimulus manipulation required. For example, pictures of two or more objects may be sufficient to evoke certain regular plural inflections, but a greater degree of verbal and concrete stimulus manipulations may be needed to evoke past tense /ed/ inflection or passive sentence forms.

Typically, the information obtained through case history, oral-peripheral examination, observations on the client's general behaviors, interviews, tests, and language samples is analyzed and integrated to obtain a total picture of the client's communicative behaviors. The case history and interview provide the background information. The tests, language samples, and other observations help determine the current communicative behaviors of the client. The test results and language samples are analyzed to find out what types of speech, language, voice, or fluency behaviors are present, and what types of behaviors are not present. For example, the phonemes the child can produce accurately may be determined along with those that cannot be produced. In terms of language, various grammatic, semantic, and pragmatic features that are present may be identified along with those that are not. Similarly, normal and abnormal voice characteristics and percentages of fluency and dysfluency rates may be determined for individual clients.

Limitations of Traditional Assessment Procedures

Traditionally, as soon as an analysis of the assessment data has been completed, the client is considered ready for intervention. Unfortunately, this is a questionable assumption because of the limitations of assessment procedures used routinely in speech-language pathology. Many of these limitations center on the concepts of reliability and validity of measures obtained during typical assessment situations. These limitations are especially noteworthy in the context of standardized tests.

Since there is no reliability without repeated measures, a single measure taken during a single assessment session does not establish reliability of the measured speech-language behaviors. Assessment is typically supposed to document the need for clinical intervention by showing that the client is not able to produce certain communicative behaviors. In order for the clinician to later demonstrate the effects of treatment or improvement in the client behaviors, the initial assessment data must be reliable. If not reliable, the need for, or the results of, clinical treatment may become questionable. For instance, in measurement of language behaviors, at least two language samples should be obtained to make sure of the presence or absence of behaviors.

Yet, it is not uncommon for treatment to be started as soon as the traditional assessment procedure has been completed.

Validity means that what is supposed to have been measured is indeed measured. In a limited sense, most tests and language samples can be considered valid because they do seem to sample speech and language behaviors. When a test appears to measure what it is supposed to measure, it is said to have face validity. It is only a superficial kind of validity, and there are other, more appropriate means of establishing validity of a measure.

The question of validity is especially serious when certain inferences are drawn from measures of communicative behaviors whose validity is not established, or is limited to face validity. On the basis of such measures, inferences may be made regarding the communicative behaviors of the client in his or her natural environments. For instance, a language sample taken in the clinic may not accurately reflect the language behaviors of the client in the home, school, or occupational setting. Additional inferences may be drawn regarding response modes that were not tested. Such inferences may also be questionable. For example, responses given on test items may not reflect conversational speech or oral reading skills. Similarly, imitative responses may not necessarily suggest productive skills.

If the purpose of an assessment is to find a client's typical communicative behaviors, then those behaviors must be sampled adequately and repeatedly. The behaviors should also be sampled in multiple settings, and in different response modes if relevant.

Other than a lack of multiple measures, most of the problems associated with the traditional assessment procedure stem from an overdependence on standardized tests. Often, assessment is equated with testing, and the ensuing report on the client is full of test results whose reliability may be unknown. The fact that the test was "standardized" does not mean that the performance of a given client is reliable. Reliability must be established for the particular measure, taken on a specific client.

Because of the problems of reliability of a given client's tested behaviors, standardized test results may not suggest appropriate target behaviors for clinical intervention. If a test cannot firmly establish the fact that the client indeed does or does not produce various types of communicative behaviors, the target behaviors will not have been identified.

Probably the most significant methodological problem with standardized tests is that they do not sample behaviors and response modes adequately. Test developers tend to point out the large number of subjects (sample) who may have been tested in the process of standardization. Such a sample may be an adequate, though local, sampling of subjects. Unfortunately, most test developers tend to ignore the issue of sampling behaviors adequately. A test of articulation, for example, may give a client one or two opportunities to produce a phoneme in a given word position (initial, medial, or final). Phonemes may not be tested, or may be tested only inadequately in conversational speech. And yet, the test results may be an important if not the sole basis of a conclusion that the child does or does not produce the tested phoneme. On a test of language, a child may be asked to produce a given grammatic morpheme in the context of one or two sentences. Whether the child does or does not produce the feature in those particular contexts may lead to the conclusion that the child is or is not able to produce that morpheme. This is often true of many aspects of language included in a variety of tests. These and other conclusions based on extremely limited sampling of behaviors are inevitable when standardized tests are relied on exclusively.

There are some equally significant philosophical problems with the use of standardized tests. First, tests encourage the use of limited and standardized stimulus materials to evoke responses. In many cases, it may be more appropriate to design stimulus materials that are appropriate to the individual client. Stimuli selected for specific clients can be more meaningful from the standpoint of training and eventual maintenance of target responses.

Second, all standardized tests are based on the concept of norms, which is the performance of a typical group. Norms are statistical averages of group performance. The performance of individuals within groups, on the other hand, typically varies to a considerable extent. But such individual variations are lost in the statistical averaging process. Thus, norms do not do justice to individual uniqueness or differences. Individual performance cannot be adequately predicted from group norms, but this difficulty in the use of test results is usually overlooked.

Assessment as Measurement of Client Behaviors

An alternative way of looking at assessment is that it is a process of measuring client behaviors. Unlike the medical model, assessment or diagnostics rarely involves the discovery of the instigating (original) cause of the speech-language disorder in given clients. Before the treatment is started, the clinician needs to determine the current communicative behaviors of the client, and this is the accepted function of an assessment. This can be achieved by measuring those behaviors. In obtaining reliable and valid measurement of communicative behaviors, the following four criteria can be useful.

First, all of the relevant response modes must be measured. Measures of imitative and evoked ("spontaneous") behaviors must be obtained. Also, conversational speech and, whenever appropriate, oral reading modes should be measured. In most cases, response topography (form of a response) should be considered also. For example, the rate of stuttering or correct production of phonemes must be measured at the levels of single words, phrases, and sentences.

Second, the behaviors to be measured must be sampled adequately. Whether it is a client's articulation, language, stuttering, or some characteristics of voice, the number of observations must be sufficient to establish reliability. In the assessment of articulation, phonemes must be tested with multiple words, phrases, and sentences. Several opportunities must be given for each position in which the phonemes are tested. Language structures should also be evaluated with multiple linguistic contexts. For example, if the present progressive /ing/ is to be tested, it must be presented in the context of at least 15 to 20 words, phrases, or sentences. The rate of stuttering must be measured with extended conversational speech and oral reading samples. Vocal behaviors (voice characteristics) must also be measured with extended speech samples, oral reading samples, or both.

Third, all measurements must be repeated to establish the reliability of measures obtained on a given client. The fact that the measurement procedures used by the clinician, such as standardized tests, were reliable with some other subjects is no basis for concluding that the given client behaviors were also measured reliably. The relevant behaviors must be measured on at least two occasions. If the two measures do not agree, additional measures must be obtained. The basic requirement is that across two or more measures, the behavior being measured meets some criterion of stability. Criteria used are more or less stringent, depending upon the purposes of the measurement. In most cases, a criterion of no more than 2 percent variation in behaviors across two measures can be adequate. It is better to use a specified criterion consistently.

Fourth, it is very desirable to obtain measures of behaviors in extraclinical situations, since reliability must be established across settings. In view of the importance of generalization and maintenance of trained behaviors, it is useful to obtain pretreatment measures of behaviors in nonclinical situations. This is probably the most difficult of the measurement requirements, since it needs the cooperation of parents and other persons involved in those situations. It also means that the clinician must go to those situations to measure behaviors, or train either the client or the parents to record them. In many cases, it is possible to have the clients or parents simply tape-record language samples at home and submit them for evaluation by the clinician. In Chapter 9 we shall discuss in some detail the issue of parent training designed to accomplish these and other objectives.

Within the traditional assessment format, it is usually not possible to measure the target behaviors according to the four criteria specified here. In any assessment, the clinician will have barely sufficient time to take the history, interview the client or the parents, do the oral-peripheral examination, administer selected tests, if any, and take conversational and (if appropriate) oral reading samples. Detailed measurement as just described takes time. Consequently, the typical assessment can only help identify a range of potential target behaviors that need to be measured further. Even this limited purpose can be better served if the clinician does not spend most of the assessment time in administering standardized tests. Extended observations, conversational speech-language samples, and simple interactions will be more useful in identifying behaviors that must be measured in some detail. Then, before the treatment is started, a limited number of potential target behaviors can be selected and measured appropriately. These pretreatment measures of target behaviors, called baselines, are described in Chapter 4.

SELECTION OF TARGET BEHAVIORS

The need to select target behaviors stems from two considerations. First, most clients with communicative disorders need treatment on multiple targets. A majority of children with articulation disorders need training on more than one phoneme. Typically, language disordered children are not able to produce a variety of language behaviors, described as grammatic, semantic, or pragmatic structures, or different classes of verbal behaviors. Some clients may have more than one kind of communicative disorder. A child, for example, may misarticulate multiple phonemes and not produce several structures of language. A child with a repaired cleft may have articulation problems along with some voice disorders of resonance. In each of these cases, the clinician must make a judgment as to which behaviors are treated, and in what sequence.

Second, in case of several disorders, theoretical considerations dictate the selection of certain target behaviors for training. In the treatment of stuttering, for example, an almost endless variety of target behaviors has been used over the centuries. Some of the behaviors targeted for training in modern times include self-confidence, self-image, anxiety, muscular tension, psychosexual aberrations, psychological role conflict, faulty attitudes, motor integration, "fluent" stuttering, rhythmic speech, reduced rate, gentle phonatory onset, prolonged speech, and regulated breathing. To a certain extent, the actual target selected for treatment depends on the theory of stuttering adopted by the clinician.

In the area of language disorders, too, researchers with differing theoretical viewpoints have advocated different targets for training. Over the years, clinicians have been asked to train auditory and visual processing, comprehension of spoken language, rules of grammar, syntactic and morphologic features, semantic concepts, pragmatic structures, and response classes. In the treatment of articulation disorders, targets such as auditory discrimination, isolated practice of sounds, production of phonemes in nonsense syllables or meaningful speech, distinctive features, and phonological rules or processes have all been suggested as treatment targets.

It is obvious that when theories change, the target behaviors also change. When language was viewed from the standpoint of universal transformational grammar, the advocated clinical targets were the rules of grammar. When the theoretical emphasis shifted from grammar to meaning, semantic features were the recommended treatment targets. When the theory shifted again from semantics to pragmatics, rules of language usage were considered more appropriate targets. Similar changes in the study of articulation have resulted in shifting target behaviors. The trend is perhaps common to most if not all disorders of communication.

A Practical Approach to the Selection of Target Behaviors

Shifting theories sometimes suggest scientific progress, and the clinician should be able to change the target behaviors accordingly. However, theoretical shifts do not always suggest advances in the study of a subject matter. Many "new" viewpoints may turn out to be short-lived from both a theoretical and a practical standpoint. In just a few years, there have been several "revolutions" in the study of language. The frequency of changes suggests that new theories were premature, could not be sustained by research, and therefore were discarded in a hurry. Sometimes new theories seem to die down only to be revived again after some years. Frequently advanced "new" theories in the field of stuttering testify to this trend. Such frequent "revolutions," changes, and shifts in emphasis create an ever-changing bandwagon effect. Many clinicians who earnestly wish to keep abreast of changes may find themselves climbing somewhat bewildered onto such bandwagons almost as frequently as getting off of them.

What the clinician needs is a practical and nontheoretical approach to the selection of target behaviors. The approach should be based not on speculative and theoretical reasoning but on clinical and experimental research. The approach should be flexible enough to accommodate changing viewpoints that are experimentally based and clinically verified. At the same time, it should be based on long accepted, repeatedly tested principles, so that inconsequential shifts in emphasis and viewpoints do not undermine clinical practice.

It is suggested here that an approach based on the concepts and methods of an experimental science will fulfill these requirements. Experimental clinical research has shown that it is possible to identify target behaviors in a nontheoretical way so that different kinds of target behaviors, as long as they are clinically proved, can be formulated. The concept of response classes provides a means of identifying target behaviors in this manner.

RESPONSE CLASSES AS TARGET BEHAVIORS

Target behaviors selected for clinical intervention must be empirically valid. In everyday language, that means that the target behaviors must be real. When put to empirical test, some of the behaviors categorized purely on theoretical grounds may turn out to be invalid. The same thing can happen when behaviors are categorized according to their structures. Linguistic analysis of language takes this approach. Syntactic, morphologic, semantic, and pragmatic aspects are based on structural analysis of language. In identifying a category of language response such as pronouns or prepositions, what is taken into consideration is the form of responses. Similarly, a question or a passive sentence is identified on the basis of the structure of those utterances. If an utterance takes one shape, it belongs to one linguistic category, and if it takes another shape, it belongs to another category.

Purely structural analysis can suggest responses that are unreal because it does not take into account the independent variables of those responses. The problem arises because the structural analysis is not sensitive to the possibility that (1) behaviors with the same structure or form may have different independent variables and that (2) behaviors with different structures may have the same independent variables. This possibility has been verified and supported by clinical research, which has also suggested a better way of conceptualizing target behaviors in terms of response classes.

A few examples will illustrate the concept of response class and the limitations of the structural analysis. First, take the example of the plural as a grammatic feature. The common linguistic analysis classifies the plural feature into two categories: the regular and the irregular. Accordingly, if a language delayed child does not produce the plural, then the clinician has those two features to train. However, when some clinicians trained the regular plural with /s/ inflections, they found out that the clients overgeneralized it to plural words with /z/ inflections (see Guess and Baer, 1973). It was then necessary to train the regular plural /z/ separately. Furthermore, other "allomorphic variations" (/əz/ as in dresses and /vəz/ as in leaves) of the regular plural were also to be trained separately. Thus, although the structural analysis had suggested one target behavior in terms of the "regular plural," in reality there were several target behaviors, each corresponding to an allomorphic variation of the grammatic morpheme.

An absence of the irregular plural, which according to the structural theory is a single category, suggests a single target behavior. But if a client needs training on the irregular plural, the clinician really does not have a single response category, but as many categories as there are irregular plurals in the English language (Hegde and McConn, 1981). For instance, a client taught to produce such words as *women, men,* and *children* will not come up with generalized (untrained) productions of other irregular plurals such as *teeth* or *feet.*

The past tense also poses similar problems. The regular past tense inflection breaks into several independent target behaviors, depending upon whether the inflected word ends with a /d/ (as in *buzzed*), or a /t/ (as in *baked*), or with an /ed/ (as in *counted*). In addition, each irregular past tense is also a unique target behavior to be trained separately. These examples make it clear that a single grammatic category may turn into a collection of different target behaviors, each in need of separate training.

Clinical research has also documented those behaviors that are considered separate within the structural analysis, but are indeed the same empirically. First, take the example of subject noun and object noun phrases. McReynolds and Engmann (1974) selected some children who did not produce either the subject noun phrase or the object noun phrase. The children were then trained in the production of subject noun phrases. Without any training whatsoever, the subjects began to produce the object noun phrases as well. The experimental control was established within a reversal design, described in Chapter 2. In essence, their results demonstrated that subject noun and object noun phrases are not separate target behaviors, as is suggested by the structural theory of grammar.

A second example of structurally different but empirically the same response category can be found in the distinction between verbal auxiliary and copula. A study by Hegde (1980) has demonstrated that when children who produce neither auxiliary *is* nor copula *is* are trained to produce only one of them, the other untrained feature may be produced without specific training. A study by Hegde and McConn (1981) obtained similar results with the auxiliary *are* and copula *are*. In both of these studies, extraneous independent variables were controlled within a reversal design. Again, what were considered to be different responses within a structural anlaysis turned out to be the same in clinical research.

The clinical research designed to identify true response classes in normal and disordered language is still in its early stages. Most of the studies have been concerned with grammatic features. With regard to semantic concepts and pragmatic structures or rules, the concept of response classes has not been researched from a clinical training standpoint. Besides, the basic semantic and pragmatic analyses have not been experimental in the sense of isolating independent variables of hypothesized response categories. Therefore, categories identified in those analyses may or may not have empirical validity.

There are just a few studies on response classes in articulation disorders and stuttering. In recent years, the study of articulation has also become very structurally oriented. This is illustrated by the distinctive feature theories and the more recent phonological theories. In either of these theories, responses are grouped according to their topographic (form-related) characteristics. There is not enough experimental evidence to show that all sounds sharing common distinctive features belong to the same response class or that sounds not sharing features belong to different classes.

Currently popular phonologic processes present similar difficulties. It is not clear that different phonological processes are systematically related to empirical response classes. For example, processes such as cluster reductions and final consonantal deletions (Compton, 1970; Ingram, 1976) may not be anything more than rational constructs. If cluster reduction is a general response class, then training on a few clusters should eliminate all other cluster reduction problems in a given client. Clinical-experimental evidence does not support this possibility, however (McReynolds and Elbert, 1981). It is possible that under experimental scrutiny, responses grouped under a process or a distinctive feature may turn out to be independent of each other. It is also possible that some of the multitudes of features and processes may collapse into fewer empirically valid response classes.

In the case of stuttering, the question is whether different forms of dysfluencies, (such as part-word repetitions, interjections, and prolongations) and associated motor behaviors (such as an eye blink) belong to the same or different response classes. Although there are some conflicting results (Brutten, 1975), the bulk of the evidence suggests that most forms of dysfluencies of stutterers belong to the same response class (Ingham, 1984). It is quite possible that associated motor behaviors of stutterers also belong to the same response class, although this question has not been researched adequately.

What are Response Classes?

Responses that have the same or similar antecedents and consequences form a class. To put it differently, a response class is a group of responses created by the same contingency or similar contingencies. If this is true, it is the clinician, not the theorist or the structuralist, who has the best chance of discovering response classes. In working with a client, the clinician typically selects a response for training, arranges antecedents (stimulus conditions) for that response, and programs certain consequences such as reinforcers and punishers.

When a few of the responses from a given class (known or unknown) are established in this manner, the client may begin to produce other responses from the same class without additional training. This happens because of generalization. The clinician will then have identified a class of responses that shared the same contingency.

An example follows. A clinician wishing to train the production of the auxiliary *is* in a language disordered child selects several sentences in which that feature is used (Hegde, 1980). Some of these sentences are then trained with appropriate stimulus conditions and response consequences (contingencies). After training a few sentences, the clinician might present the remaining untrained sentences to see whether the auxiliary *is* is generalized. Assuming that the amount of training was adequate, the child might produce the target feature in those untrained sentences. Then all of the trained and untrained sentences with the auxiliary *is* would belong to a single response class. If as a result, the child begins to produce the copula *is* as well, then the production of copula is under the control of the same contingency that created the production of auxiliary *is*. This possibility would be strengthened when the copula is trained and the auxiliary is produced without additional training. If such results are obtained with appropriate controls (such as reversal of contingencies), a single response class, including both auxiliary and copula, will have been identified. That these two are treated as different in structural analysis (grammar) would be irrelevant to clinical intervention strategies.

Response classes can be identified only by experimental research in which antecedents and consequences are manipulated. Linguistic analysis is typically nonexperimental. As such, it identifies response categories on a rational basis. Such categories may or may not hold up under experimental scrutiny. The clinician who selects linguistically based categories of semantics, grammar, and pragmatics for the target behaviors is taking a certain amount of risk. Some of those categories may not contain empirical responses at all, and a certain other category may be more than a single response entity. The problem then is that the clinician would not know the number of target behaviors that need clinical training. A given feature (plural /s/, for example) may be more than one target, and two features (auxiliary and copula) may be actually a single target. Therefore, clinicians should determine what to train by clinical research.

Clinicians who can determine response classes by experimental-clinical research will be basing their target behaviors on the methods and concepts of scientific experimentation. The experimental procedure involved in the identification of response classes is not limited by a particular theory. If new response categories are suggested by nonexperimental research, the clinician can put them to experimental test. Any structural or other kind of category that proves to be empirically real can be a target behavior.

Unfortunately, many target behaviors (semantic concepts, pragmatic rules, distinctive features, phonological processes) that have been suggested in recent years have not been experimentally tested. It is known that many of the grammatic features may not be empirically valid. It would be helpful if the tendency to categorize behaviors on the basis of their structures is tempered by the experimental method.

It can be expected that continued research on response classes will be able to identify empirically valid clinical target behaviors. Even then, there would be a need to select target behaviors. As stated earlier, most clients need training on multiple targets and only a few of them can be trained at any given time. Therefore, with most clients, the clinician is likely to face the problem of the selection of target behaviors.

A problem closely related to the selection of target behaviors concerns the sequence in which multiple targets should be trained. Multiple responses can be trained in one of several different sequences, and what sequence to follow is a question the clinician needs to answer. There are two approaches to these interrelated problems of selection and training sequence; one is based on normative information, and the other on individual-specific considerations.

THE NORMATIVE STRATEGY

Clinicians have traditionally used the normative strategy in determining both the target behaviors and the sequence in which they are trained. Of course, this strategy is most relevant to disorders of language and articulation in which multiple target behaviors are typically selected and trained on the basis of normative information.

It is generally believed that clinical training must follow the sequence found in normally developing children. Behaviors that are normally mastered earlier in the sequence are supposed to be taught before those that are mastered later. Studies of normal language acquisition are supposed to have established norms that specify ages at which children master different grammatic, semantic, or pragmatic features. The normative studies are also supposed to have determined the sequence in which various language behaviors are acquired. Once this information is available, the clinician is thought to be in a position to determine the target behaviors and their sequence of training. If the client is a four year old child, then the sequential norms for four year olds will dictate the targets and the treatment sequence.

The normative strategy is probably one of the most widely accepted clinical strategies in speech-language pathology. A closer examination of this strategy, however, raises certain troublesome questions that have important clinical consequences. These questions are related to three basic assumptions inherent to the normative strategy. The first is that there are age-based norms, which can help with decisions regarding individual clients. The second is that there is a fixed sequence in which language behaviors are learned by most if not all children. The third is that the sequence found in normally developing children is the best sequence to use in clinical training. Each of these assumptions deserves careful consideration.

Are There Valid and Useful Age-Based Norms?

By definition, norms refer to the performance of a typical group. What is a typical group, and whether it has been adequately sampled in establishing norms, are two critical questions in this regard. Most frequently, norms are established with the method of cross-sectional sampling of a group of children. Such norms are more likely to be established by those who wish to construct tests of speech and language behaviors. When a new test of articulation or language development is being constructed, it is administered to a sample of children at selected age levels. The performance of children in the study becomes the norm for the age groups sampled.

Norms are rarely established on a large enough sample to make them representative of children seen in clinics across the country. At best, they may be local norms relevant to children in the area sampled. Even then, because of practical problems, samples are not always drawn strictly according to the random procedure. Therefore, to what extent the performance of the sampled children represents the performance of unselected children in the local or distant areas may remain doubtful.

There is a different kind of problem with norms even when they are based on samples drawn randomly from a large population. This problem arises because norms are a statistical representation of the mean (average) performance of the entire group. As noted before, the mean usually does not reflect an individual subject's performance accurately. Variations in individual performance will have been masked by the mean. As a result, the clinician cannot use norms to determine the particular communicative behaviors of a given child. Indeed, the larger the sample, and hence the more representative it is of the population, the less relevant the results to predicting the individual performance. This is because very large samples will also have included subjects of varied social, educational, and personal backgrounds, with the result that a given individual's performance is likely to be even more different from the statistical mean.

The fact that norms have not yet been established for several aspects of communicative behaviors is often considered a major problem for the clinician. However, in view of these problems associated with norms, it appears that the lack of norms is not as handicapping as the basic concept itself.

Another method can provide more useful information than statistical norms. This method involves repeated observations on a single child or a few children. Brown's (1973) now classic study of three children's language learning process illustrates this method. Language samples are recorded periodically, and the changes in the children's responses over time are analyzed. This is the well-known longitudinal method. There are only a few studies of this kind because they are expensive and time-consuming. Since a few children are studied intensively, individual variations and unique patterns are readily recognized. This type of information can be more useful than the statistical mean when the clinician is trying to understand the communicative behaviors of particular children. Since the longitudinal method typically involves a small number of subjects, they are less likely to yield statistical norms of language development. Instead, they focus upon the sequence with which some subjects learn different language behaviors, which leads us to the second assumption of the normative strategy.

Is There a Fixed Sequence of Language Acquisition?

The question of sequence of acquisition is more often debated in the context of language, but the basic logic applies to all aspects of communicative behaviors. The assumption that there is a sequence in which children normally learn communicative behaviors is about as widely accepted as the concept of norms. Any statement regarding the existence of a sequence in language learning can be more or less controversial, depending on how the statement is interpreted. If the statement refers to a broad and variable pattern in learning language, it is probably least controversial. By and large, children tend to master certain responses before they learn certain other responses. However, if this is interpreted to mean that the sequence is invariable across children (Brown, 1974; Dale, 1976; de Villiers and de Villiers, 1973), and that there may be an innate mechanism that universally determines the sequence, then the statement is highly questionable. Known sequences of language acquisition are not invariable, and some sequences may simply be due to the nature of language. For example, the child has no use for an auxiliary *is* until the present progressive *ing* is learned. Some of the language "structures" may be elements of a chain, but different elements may be acquired at different times. More importantly, most of the sequences researched so far have shown individual differences.

Even if certain sequences do exist, there is no assurance that a sequence is a product of inferred mental variables such as innate mechanisms and cognitive stages. Known sequences in behaviors do not automatically rule out the influence of external (manipulable) independent variables. It is possible that by control of those independent variables, the sequence of behavior acquisition can be altered. What is needed is experimental research on the acquisition of communicative behaviors in children. Mere observational technique, which is so commonly used in the study of language, does not support or refute hypotheses concerning the manipulability of observed sequences or patterns. There is some experimental evidence that children who are learning the language normally can be taught grammatic structures out of their known sequences (Capelli, 1985; De Cesari, 1985; Nelson, 1977).

Should Clinical Training Follow Normative Sequences?

The third assumption of the normative strategy - that it is best to follow the developmental sequence in clinical training - is one of the most untested of the common assumptions of clinical practice. As yet, there is no convincing evidence to suggest that (1) within certain limits, a sequence other than the normative is particularly difficult to implement clinically, and (2) clients learn or generalize faster when the training is based on the normative sequence. Besides, if it is true that within limits, specific speech-language behaviors can be taught or modified by gaining control over their independent variables, then there is no compelling reason to follow the normative sequence in clinical training.

As Guess, Sailor, and Baer (1978) have pointed out, the best sequence of training must be determined by clinical research. It is possible that the sequence in which children normally learn language is indeed the best strategy to teach target behaviors to clinical populations. On the other hand, a sequence not consistent with normative information may be just as effective, or even more so. The issue then must be addressed by controlled clinical research in which different sequences are systematically evaluated to see which ones are more efficient. Clinicians should feel free to experiment with different sequences and carefully record the results of such manipulations. In essence, better sequences in which target behaviors are trained will be determined not by identifying the normal sequence, but by clinical experimentation with different sequences.

Because of its fundamental philosophical assumptions, the normative strategy is unlikely to encourage experimentation with different sequences in which the target behaviors can be trained. What is needed is a strategy that is free from the assumptions of the normative approach and that can permit clinical experimentation.

THE CLIENT-SPECIFIC STRATEGY

An alternative to the normative strategy can be called the client-specific strategy; it is based on the philosophy that the selection of target behaviors as well as the sequence in which they are trained must be client-specific. The normative information can provide some broad guidelines but can hardly suggest specific target behaviors. Within this philosophy, the justification for the actual target behaviors selected for treatment must be based on the individual client's particular situation, not statistical norms (Guess et al., 1978). In the selection of target behaviors for a given client, factors such as the client's environment, the relevance or usefulness of the behaviors selected, the potential for generalization and maintenance, and the potential for behavioral expansion are considered.

Within the client-specific strategy, before the target behaviors are selected, the client's particular environment is studied to determine what kinds of behavioral demands are placed upon that client. Age-specific norms play only a minor role, if at all, in the selection process. For example, a ten year old child in need of clinical services may be "functioning more like a six year old," to use a typical expression, but this may not necessarily mean that the target behaviors should be the typical (if known) behaviors of a six year old. In many ways, the ten year old child might be different from most six year olds. The child may be in a special educational program whose demands may be different from those faced by normal six year olds. At home and on the playground, the child may be expected to do things other than what would be expected of a six year old. The client's physical development may be far ahead of the language behaviors, which might also lead to different kinds of demands on the child. In situations such as these, it may be more appropriate to select target behaviors that are specific to the particular client. The selected behaviors may or may not bear a specific relation to the norms.

The need to study the client's environment becomes even more obvious with adult mentally retarded subjects whose speech and language behaviors are below their age levels. It is probably least appropriate to select the typical language behaviors of a ten year old because the retarded adult client's "language age" is ten years. It is possible that this client is working in a sheltered workshop or in a special job training program. The best speech-language services for such clients are not the age-based normative behaviors, but the particular kinds of language that can make them more efficient in their occupational or educational situations. In determining the target behaviors, an analysis of the sheltered workshop situation or the job training program would be more appropriate than checking out the norms. It may be better to teach the client the vocabulary and the language responses used in those particular situations. Aphasic adults who have lost speech to varying degrees are in similar situations. That the client has lost most of his speech and thus resembles a child in terms of language behaviors does not mean that the target behaviors should be selected on the basis of the client's "functional age."

The second consideration is that the language behaviors taught must be useful or relevant to the client (Guess et al., 1978). Several target behaviors typically taught in clinical situations may not be useful to the clients at all. Routine selection of target responses that label color, shape, and size illustrate behaviors that have very little usefulness to the client. A child going around the house naming colors and identifying shapes and sizes of objects is not exhibiting relevant verbal behavior. In some cases, even counting numbers and reciting days of the week and months of the year may not be very useful. As suggested by Guess and co-worker,(1978), the most useful behaviors may be those that give the client a means of controlling his or her environment. A child who is able to say "juice please" can exert more precise control over others than the one who points to the refrigerator. Mands (commands, demands, requests) that result in specific reinforcement for the client are more useful than some other kinds of target behaviors. The child who is able to ask for things needed, tell about personal experiences, and indicate internal states of pain and motivation has a more effective repertoire of verbal behavior than a child who can only name colors or recite days of the week.

The third consideration is that the target behaviors must have a potential for generalization and maintenance. Traditionally, generalization and maintenance were thought to be a matter to be considered only after the target behaviors were established. However, some clinical research suggests that the clinician needs to think of generalization and maintenance even before the target behaviors are selected. This is so because some target behaviors may generalize and be maintained more readily than other behaviors. Generally speaking, behaviors that are useful to the client and are likely to be exhibited in the natural environment may have a better chance of becoming initially generalized to the client's everyday situations. Once generalized, those responses are more likely to come under the influence of reinforcing contingencies at home. When this happens, the chances of response maintenance are enhanced. We shall discuss the generalization and maintenance strategies in Chapter 7.

The fourth consideration is that the behaviors to be trained must serve as building blocks for new behaviors that the client can produce without additional training. This potential for behavioral expansion can be called response generalization or induction. It means that untrained and more complex responses can be produced without further teaching. When mastered, various grammatic features permit response induction. For example, a child taught to use the copula *is* in the context of the personal pronoun *he* ("he is good") may be able to produce that copula in the context of other pronouns, such as *she* ("she is nice"). Similarly, a client taught to produce the possessive inflection in the context of a given set of nouns ("man's paper," "man's hat") may be able to produce the inflection in the context of other nouns, such as "lady's hat" and "lady's purse" (Hegde, Noll, and Pecora, 1979).

Some types of responses may be limited in terms of response expansion. Simple labeling of objects or colors and routine responses like reciting the days of the week, or questions like "What is that?" may be so limited. This does not mean that such responses should not be taught at all, but that when they are taught, their limitations should be considered. Additional behaviors with better potential for response induction must be taught before the client's conditioned repertoire can be expected to expand.

In summary, clinicians have typically adopted the normative strategy in the selection of target behaviors. This strategy has certain limitations that are both philosophical and methodological. An alternative strategy involves client-specific considerations. In selecting the target behaviors, the clinician should consider the environment of the client, the usefulness of the behaviors, the potential for generalization and maintenance, and response expansion possibilities.

DEFINITION OF TARGET BEHAVIORS

Selection and definition of target behaviors are interrelated. Initially, the selected target behaviors may be identified in general terms. Soon, the behaviors must be defined in precise terms. There are several reasons why the target behaviors must be defined in certain ways. First, in order to be accountable, the clinician must measure the target behaviors before, during, and after treatment. This continuous process of measurement becomes possible only when the responses are defined precisely. Vague definitions do not permit objective measurements. Second, objective definitions allow other clinicians to replicate the treatment in teaching the same target behaviors to other clients. Third, objective definitions make it possible for an external observer to verify the results of clinical services. For these and other reasons, it is necessary to define target behaviors in an appropriate manner.

Essentially, there are two ways of defining target behaviors: constituent and operational. The most important distinction between the two is that constituent definitions may not suggest procedures of measurement, whereas operational definitions do.

Constituent Definitions

Constituent definitions are also called conceptual definitions. These come close to everyday definitions of words. Dictionaries often use constituent definitions. They are essentially definitions of terms with the help of other terms that refer to other concepts. If the meaning of these other concepts is not known, the definitions may not help. For example, to define language as linguistic competence is to define that term constituently. If the meaning of linguistic competence is not clear, then the definition is not helpful. But more importantly, the definition does not say how language can be measured. As another example, to define intelligence as mental capacity is to define it constituently. The term mental capacity may be just as vague as intelligence, and therefore may not permit measurement. If stuttering is defined as a disorder of rhythm, one must know normal and disordered rhythm before the definition can make any sense. Similarly, an articulation disorder may be defined conceptually as an inability to acquire phonological rules, but before this definition can be used in measurement, it must go through a series of translations.

Constituent definitions not only are used in describing disorders and general behaviors, but also are often used in defining specific responses targeted for clinical intervention. For example, the treatment target for a language disordered child may be defined as "linguistic competence." But this definition does not specify how the behavior can be measured to show that the client who did not have that target began to show it after treatment. Another clinician may define the goal of an articulation treatment program as teaching phonological rules, but this definition does not specify how to demonstrate whether the client has or has not learned those rules. Other treatment goals may be defined as an increased level of self-confidence, better self-image, increased communicative competence, stimulation of language abilities, facilitation of communicative behaviors, enrichment of language, and so on. Each of these target behaviors (treatment goals) make conceptual sense, or so it is generally thought. But they do not tell the clinician how to measure those behaviors.

Operational Definitions

Operational definitions are those that define behaviors in terms of measurement procedures. In a sense, operational definitions are really not definitions per se. They are more like descriptions of operations that are necessary to measure behaviors being defined. A clinician who comes across an operational definition should be able to measure the behavior by simply following the descriptions. To take an extreme example, intelligence may be defined as a persons's score on the Stanford-Binet test of intelligence. In order to determine a person's intelligence, all you have to do is to administer the Stanford-Binet test and score the performance according to the standard procedure. A child's language behavior may be defined as his or her score on a particular language test, although we do not have such a comprehensive test available. As will be shown shortly, behaviors can be defined operationally without the help of test results.

Operational definitions are probably more useful in specifying clinical targets than in describing behaviors at a global and theoretical level. Clinical targets usually have limited scope. A clinician wishing to train the "language competence" of a client would probably have a very long way to travel, and would not know when and whether the destination had been reached. Therefore, treatment targets are more narrowly defined so that they can be observed and measured.

Training considerations also require that the target responses be limited in scope, narrowly defined, and observable. A well defined response of limited scope has a better potential of being trained than a global language competence or communicative ability. In addition, the clinician can manipulate only a few independent (treatment) variables at a time. Therefore, at any given time, only a few specific dependent (response) variables can be handled efficiently. Several examples of operational definitions can be considered. In the treatment of a child who is minimally verbal, certain words can be selected as the target behaviors. The treatment target can be defined as "the production of the following ten words at 90 percent accuracy when asked to name appropriate pictures across two consecutive sessions" and include a list of the selected words.

If the training is expected to involve morphologic features, then the treatment targets can be specified in terms of selected morphemes. For example, the target behavior may be defined as "the production of the regular plural morpheme /s/ at the level of single words while naming 20 pictures with 90 percent accuracy." Eventually, the plural morpheme may be trained at the level of conversational speech. Then the target behavior may be redefined as "the production of the regular plural morpheme /s/ in conversational speech at 90 percent accuracy across two consecutive sessions each with a minimum of 20 opportunities to produce the target behavior." The final or the dismissal criterion may be defined as "the production of the regular plural morpheme /s/ in conversational speech exhibited in the child's home at 90 percent accuracy across two separate language samples, with each sample containing at least 20 opportunities for the morpheme production." These examples make it clear that the target behaviors are defined somewhat differently depending upon the level of training.

If treatment involves certain syntactic formulation, the targets may be defined as "the production of three to four word sentences in conversational speech across three home samples each containing at least 100 utterances." Various syntactic structures can then be specified in the description of the treatment targets.

The treatment targets in the area of articulation disorders are also narrowly defined. Typically, the speech sounds are trained in the initial, medial, and final positions of words. For example, the phoneme /s/ may be trained in words such as *sun* and *soup* (initial), *muscle* and *hassle* (medial), and *toss* and *boss* (final). The initial treatment target for a given child may be defined as "the correct production of /s/ in the initial position of words evoked on a set of 20 discrete trials at 90 percent accuracy." A subsequent treatment target may be defined as "the correct production of /s/ in the initial position of words used in two-word phrases evoked on a set of 20 discrete trials at 90 percent accuracy." Similar definitions would be required at the level of sentences and conversational speech. The final dismissal criterion may be defined as the "correct production of /s/ in conversational speech at home and other situations at 90 percent accuracy across three language samples each containing a minimum of 20 opportunities for the production of /s/." Production of sounds in the medial and final position of words can be similarly defined.

In the treatment of stuttering, it is probably necessary to distinguish the eventual outcome of the treatment program and the specific target behaviors that must be trained in order to achieve that outcome. The outcome of a stuttering treatment program can be defined as a "reduction in dysfluencies to less than 1 percent in conversational speech in clinical settings, and no more than 5 percent in everyday situations." The definition may also specify the length of speech samples in which the fluency is measured (e.g., 300 word samples). Alternatively, the outcome may be defined as "99 or 95 percent fluency in conversational speech." As in the treatment of any other communicative disorders, the initial, intermediate, and final outcome must be defined separately. The initial outcome in the modification of stuttering may be a "fluency rate of 99 percent or better at the level of single word responses, or during oral reading of isolated words." In either mode, fluency must be measured in multiple and consecutive samples. As the response complexity increases from the single word level to phrases and sentences, additional definitions would be required.

In most stuttering treatment programs, the operationally defined treatment outcome is achieved by training specific responses. Several treatment programs focus upon the following target behaviors: (1) an inhalation and slight exhalation before the production of an utterance, (2) maintenance of airflow throughout the utterance, (3) soft and gentle initiation of sound, (4) reduced rate of speech through stretching of the syllables, (5) soft articulatory contacts, and (6) normal prosodic features (Hegde, 1985). The normal prosodic features are a clinical target because the previous targets, when mastered, alter the pattern of speech. Though devoid of stuttering, this type of speech is unusually slow and monotonous. Therefore, the typical intonational patterns and socially acceptable rate must eventually be shaped. Except for the normal prosody, which is shaped in the latter stages of treatment, all of the target responses are initially trained at the level of single words or short phrases, and in successive steps the length of utterances is increased. Each of the target behaviors can be measured on discrete trials yielding a percent correct response rate.

Treatment targets in voice disorders are often defined in terms of the clinician's judgments or evaluations. Although sophisticated electronic instruments are available for monitoring various aspects of vocal production, most clinicians may not have access to such expensive equipment. Therefore, the clinician usually judges whether the client's voice is of acceptable pitch and intensity, and whether it is devoid of such qualities as harshness, hoarseness, or hypernasality. With the help of a piano or a pitch pipe, the habitual pitch of a client can be established. Once this is done, the most desirable pitch for that client can be determined by experimenting with various levels of pitch. Such a desirable pitch then becomes the treatment target for that client. The target itself can then be defined operationally. For example, the treatment target for a given client can be defined as "the maintenance of a level of pitch judged appropriate by the clinician with 90 percent accuracy in conversational speech exhibited in everyday situations." As with other disorders, the number and length of speech samples should also be specified.

Similar judgment-based measurement procedures can be established in treating hyper- or hypo-nasality and other vocal characteristics. An operational definition would essentially specify the absence of undesirable vocal qualities in specified speech productions evoked initially in the clinic and eventually in the client's natural environments. Also, if it is determined that certain abusive vocal habits must be changed in order to reduce undesirable vocal qualities, then the reduction in behavior becomes the treatment target. Behaviors such as excessive yelling and talking in noisy environments can be measured in terms of their frequency on a daily or weekly basis. A reduction in the number of those behavior episodes then becomes the operationally defined treatment target. For example, it may be determined that for a given child who yells too much on the playground, the treatment target may be defined as "an absence of yelling in a 30 minute play activity." If a client is known to visit noisy bars very frequently, a reduction in such visits, measured weekly, can be the treatment target.

The Five Criteria of Operational Definitions

The examples just given illustrate the basic concepts underlying operational definitions of target behaviors. An operational definition should fulfill at least the following five criteria:

1. Specify the Response Topography. The topography or the form the behaviors take must be specified. The production of the present progressive *ing*, the production of /s/ or /z/, dysfluencies such as part-word repetitions, nasal resonance on nonnasal sounds, and so on describe response forms.

2. Specify the Mode of Responses. In what mode the responses will be measured must be specified. The target responses may be measured either in oral reading, conversation, imitative speech, or nonimitative (evoked, "spontaneous") productions.

3. Specify the Level of Responses. Whether the target responses will be measured at the level of single words, two-word phrases, or complex sentences must be specified. At different stages of training, targets are measured at different levels.

4. Specify the Stimulus and Setting Conditions. Under what stimulus conditions and under what environmental settings the behaviors will be measured must be described. The responses may be measured when the client is shown pictures or asked questions, in the clinical situation, at the client's natural environment, and so on.

5. Specify the Accuracy Criterion. For the most part, a 90 percent accuracy rate is used. However, some behaviors may be held to a higher criterion. In some stuttering treatment programs, dysfluencies are held to a criterion of less than 1 percent (fluency 99 percent or better). The number of consecutive observations for which the criterion is applied must also be specified (e.g., across three speech-language samples, over a set of 20 trials, in ten consecutive responses).

Limitations of Operationalism

The operational approach has certainly helped clinicians focus on specified target behaviors that can be measured in order to document changes in those behaviors. But the approach is not without its limitations. When carried to its extreme, operationalism can turn complex concepts into meaningless definitions. For example, when intelligence is defined as a person's score on a certain test, the complex concept is reduced to a number, which may not mean anything or anything important. The fact that intelligence is now operationally defined does not mean that we understand it better than we did before it was "operationalized."

Sometimes operationalism gives an air of scientific credibility to questionable concepts. It can dress up mental, essentially unobservable concepts by redefining them in "measurable" terms. That something is somehow measured does not necessarily mean the underlying concept is valid. "Attitudes" are an excellent example. There are scales of measurement that "operationalize" attitudes. The resulting statistical analyses may give an impression of a valid scientific concept because it was measured. However, such measurement procedures may not validate the concept of attitudes. Attitudes are often inferred from certain kinds of behaviors; it may be more appropriate to measure those behaviors directly.

When the operational approach is used prudently, it can serve the clinician well. In order to establish his or her accountability, the clinician needs to measure behaviors, and operational definitions make measurement possible. The operational approach can also help avoid vague descriptions of treatment procedures. To this extent, operaionalism is useful to clinicians.

SUMMARY

Assessment of clients' communicative behaviors is the first step in providing clinical services. Traditionally, assessment involves taking a case history, interviewing the client, recording a language sample, performing an oral-peripheral examination, administering standardized tests, and conducting a closing interview. The traditional assessment tends to overemphasize the use of standardized tests. Tests have limited value because of such drawbacks as questionable statistical notions of norms, lack of reliability of measures, and limited sampling of behaviors.

Assessment is better defined as reliable and valid measurement of clients' communicative behaviors. During the assessment, (1) all response modes must be measured, (2) the behaviors must be sampled adequately, (3) all measures must be repeated, and (4) preferably, extraclinical measures must be obtained.

Multiple target behaviors and theoretical considerations create a need for selecting target behaviors. Structural categories are often selected as treatment targets. A better alternative is to select clinically verified response classes. Responses that have the same or similar antecedents and consequences form a class.

The normative and the client-specific are the two approaches to the selection of target behaviors. The client-specific strategy suggests that the client's environment, the relevance of the behaviors, the potential for maintenance, and the potential for response expansion must be considered in selecting target behaviors.

Target behaviors can be defined either constituently or operationally. The former does not specify measurement procedures, but the latter does. In defining the target behaviors operationally, the clinician must specify (1) the response topography, (2) the mode of responses, (3) the level of responses, (4) the stimulus and setting conditions, and (5) the accuracy criterion.

STUDY GUIDE

Define, describe, or answer the following questions in technical language. When you are not sure, reread the text, and when necessary, rewrite the answers.

1. Describe the traditional approach to assessment.
2. What is the recommended definition of assessment?
3. What was emphasized in the recommended assessment procedure?
4. Describe the need for selecting target behaviors.
5. What are norms?
6. Define reliability and validity.
7. Describe the language sampling procedure.
8. What are some of the things you should not do while taking a language sample from a child?
9. What are the limitations of traditional assessment procedures?
10. What are the four criteria of measurement?
11. Distinguish between subject and behavior sampling.
12. What are the limitations of standardized tests?
13. How are theories related to the selection of target behaviors?

14. What is the normative strategy?
15. Describe the client-specific strategy of selecting target behaviors.
16. What are the questionable assumptions of the normative strategy?
17. What are response classes? How are they determined?
18. Why should you be concerned with the sequence of training?
19. How should you determine the best sequence of training?
20. Describe two language response classes that do not correspond with structural (grammatic) categories.
21. What are structural categories? What critical variable is missing in pure structural analysis?
22. What are constituent definitions?
23. What are operational definitions?
24. Operationally define target behaviors for a client in the following categories:
    • Language
    • Articulation
    • Fluency
    • Voice
    • Manual signs
25. What are the two limitations of operationalism?

REFERENCES

Brutten, G. J. (1975). Stuttering: Topography, assessment, and behavior change strategies. In J. Eisenson (Ed.), *Stuttering: A second symposium* (pp. 199–262). New York: Harper and Row.

Brown, R. (1973). *A first language: The early stages.* Cambridge, MA: Harvard University Press.

Capelli, R. (1985). *An experimental analysis of morphologic acquisition.* Unpublished master's thesis, California State University, Fresno.

Compton, A. J. (1970). Generative studies of children's phonological disorders. *Journal of Speech and Hearing Disorders, 35,* 315–339.

Dale, P. S. (1976). *Language development: Structure and function.* New York: Holt, Rinehart and Winston.

Darley, F. L., and Spriestersbach, D. C. (1978) (Eds.), *Diagnostic methods in speech pathology* (2nd ed.) New York: Harper and Row.

De Cesari, R. (1985). *Experimental training of grammatic morphemes: Effects on the order of acquisition.* Unpublished master's thesis, California State University, Fresno.

de Villiers, J. G., and de Villiers, P. A. (1973). A cross-sectional study of the acquisition of grammatical morphemes in child speech. *Journal of Psycholinguistic Research, 2,* 267–278.

Guess, D. and Baer, D. M. (1973). Some experimental analyses of linguistic development in institutionalized retarded children. In B. B. Lahey (Ed.), *The modification of language behavior* (pp. 3–60). Springfield, IL: Charles C Thomas.

Guess, D., Sailor, W., and Baer, D. M. (1978). Children with limited language. In R. L. Schiefelbusch (Ed.), *Language intervention strategies* (pp. 101–143). Baltimore: University Park Press.

Hegde, M. N. (1980). An experimental-clinical analysis of grammatical and behavioral distinctions between verbal auxiliary and copula. *Journal of Speech and Hearing Research, 23,* 864–877.

Hegde, M. N. (1985). Treatment of fluency disorders: State of the art. In J. M. Costello (Ed.), *Speech disorders in adults: Recent advances* (pp.155–188). San Diego: College-Hill Press.

Hegde, M. N., and McConn, J. (1981). Language training: Some data on response classes and generalization to an occupational setting. *Journal of Speech and Hearing Disorders, 46,* 353–358.

Hegde, M. N., Noll, M. J., and Pecora, R. (1979). A study of some factors affecting generalization of language training. *Journal of Speech and Hearing Disorders, 44,* 301–320.

Ingham, R. J. (1984). *Stuttering and behavior therapy: Current status and experimental foundations.* San Diego: College-Hill Press.

Ingram, D. (1976). *Phonological disabilities in children.* New York: American Elsevier.

McReynolds, L. V. and Elbert, M. F. (1981). Generalization of correct articulation in clusters. *Applied Psycholinguistics, 2,* 119–132.

McReynolds, L. V. and Engmann, D. L. (1974). An experimental analysis of the relationship between subject noun and object noun phrases. In L. V. McReynolds (Ed.), *Developing systematic procedures for training children's language* (pp. 30–46). Rockville, MD: Asha monographs No. 18.

Nelson, K. E. (1977). Facilitating children's syntax acquisition. *Developmental Psychology, 13,* 101–107.

Peterson, H. A., and Marquardt, T. M. (1981). *Appraisal and diagnosis of speech and language disorders.* Englewood Cliffs, NJ: Prentice-Hall.

Chapter 4

Contingencies as Treatment Variables

So far, a treatment paradigm for communicative disorders has been discussed, along with techniques of documenting treatment effectiveness. In addition, procedures of selection and definition of target behaviors have also been described.

In Chapter 4, the following points will be described:

- Contingencies as treatment variables
- Positive and negative reinforcement
- Types of positive reinforcement
- Reinforcement schedules
- Use of different schedules in treatment

The professional task of the speech-language pathologist has been variously described as remediation of communicative disorders, treatment of speech-language problems, reducing communicative deficits, helping people realize their communicative potential, and so on. All of these descriptions may be appropriate, though not necessarily measurable. Essentially, they all refer to two basic tasks the speech-language pathologist typically performs.

The clinician's first basic task is to create certain kinds of communicative behaviors, increase them, or both. Clients seek professional help either because they are not able to produce certain communicative behaviors or because the behaviors are produced at very low frequency levels. A child with a language disorder may not be producing certain grammatic or semantic features or some response classes. Perhaps the child is producing those behaviors but at a very low rate. The child then needs to either learn those responses or learn to produce them more often. Similarly, a person who stutters is exhibiting less than the desirable level of fluency, and he or she wants this fluency increased. A client who cannot maintain a desirable pitch level wants this vocal behavior increased.

The clinician's second basic task is to decrease certain other behaviors that are considered undesirable by the client or society or both. This is often a counterpart of the first task of increasing desirable behaviors. A language disordered child may be using gestures that need to be decreased while verbal behaviors are increased. A stutterer's dysfluencies need to be decreased while fluency is increased. In a child with an articulation disorder, faulty production of certain speech sounds needs to be decreased while the correct production is increased. In addition, clients may exhibit interfering behaviors that are nonverbal (such as off-seat behaviors), and they too, must be reduced.

In order to be effective, the clinician needs two sets of procedures: one set to create or increase desirable target behaviors, and a second set to decrease or eliminate undesirable behaviors. From a technical standpoint, a clinician's expertise is the efficiency with which these two sets of techniques are managed. In this chapter, we shall focus upon techniques that increase behaviors that exist at a very low level. Chapter 6 is concerned with creating new behaviors and Chapter 8 with techniques of decreasing undesirable behaviors.

It was pointed out in Chapter 1 that the most significant aspect of the treatment program within the paradigm is a contingency between certain stimulus variables, a response of certain topography, and consequences arranged by the clinician. The clinician manages the interdependent relation between these three elements of the contingency. Technically speaking, the clinician-arranged response consequences are the more specific treatment variables, and a successful management of the contingency is the overall treatment.

Decades of research on human behavior has established the fact that consequences generated by responses play a very significant role in shaping the future course of those responses. More specifically, consequences determine (1) whether a response will be initially learned; (2) if it is learned, whether it will be maintained over time; and (3) the strength and frequency of maintained responses. Therefore, in teaching and learning, response consequences are extremely important. Both laboratory research and applied human research have produced extensive information on how to program response consequences so that behaviors are learned and maintained at high frequency. Basically, consequences that help learn, increase, and maintain responses are known as reinforcers. There are two kinds of reinforcers: positive and negative.

POSITIVE REINFORCERS

Positive reinforcers can be defined as those events that, when made contingent upon a response, will increase the future probability of that response. In other words, positive reinforcers are events that follow a response and thereby increase its frequency.

In order to serve as a reinforcer, an event should follow a response immediately. This is typically described as a response contingent occurrence of a consequence. A temporal gap between the response and its consequence will reduce the effectiveness of the consequence. In everyday life, consequences "naturally" follow responses. Usually, these consequences come in the form of reponses (reactions) from other people. In treatment settings, the clinician carefully selects and arranges certain consequences so that they follow the target behaviors immediately. In order to determine the actual reinforcing value of consequences, the clinician carefully monitors their effects.

In speech-language pathology, several misunderstandings prevail about the definitions of basic behavioral terms. The definitions of positive and negative reinforcers and punishment procedures are often misrepresented by both clinicians and researchers (Hegde, 1979). It is necessary to understand a few critical aspects of the definition of positive reinforcers.

First, reinforcers are not defined in terms of subjective feelings. How the clinician feels about a consequence or subjectively evaluates it is irrelevant to the definition. The clinician cannot determine that a piece of candy or verbal statements such as "excellent!" are reinforcers because people feel good about them. Giving something to a client because he or she "likes it" is no assurance that a reinforcer has been used. Such feeling states associated with reinforcers are not critical in the definition of reinforcers.

Second, whether or not a given consequence is a reinforcer is not determined beforehand. A clinician cannot say that candy will be used with client X because it is a reinforcer. It may or may not increase the client's response rate. Only after having demonstrated the positive effects of candy on client X's behavior can a clinician say that candy was used as a positive reinforcer. This means that there is no standard list of positive reinforcers from which the clinician can simply select reinforcers for given clients. There are no presumed positive reinforcers, and therefore the term is a misnomer.

Third, what is a reinforcer for one client may not be a reinforcer for another client. Indeed, a reinforcer for one client may turn out to be a punisher for another client. Therefore, it is important to determine objectively the effect of a given consequence on a particular person's rate of response. This philosophy is highly compatible with the clinical concept that each client is unique in several ways, in spite of many common characteristics across clients. Therefore, every time a clinician decides to use a certain consequence as a reinforcer with a given client, the rate of response must be measured continuously.

Fourth, what has been demonstrated to be a reinforcer in a given client at one time may or may not act as a reinforcer at another time. This also emphasizes the need to measure the response rates continuously. Obviously, all consequated responses must be objectively defined so that they can be measured precisely.

TYPES OF POSITIVE REINFORCERS

There are five main types of positive reinforcers: (1) primary, or unconditioned; (2) secondary, social, or conditioned; (3) conditioned generalized; (4) informative feedback; and (5) high probability behaviors.

Primary, or Unconditioned, Reinforcers

Some reinforcers are classified as primary, or unconditioned, because their effects do not depend upon past experience. In other words, they are not learned. Genetic and neurophysiological mechanisms of species predispose their members to react in certain ways to certain stimuli. Food is a major form of primary reinforcer. Other edible or consumable items that may or may not have a significant food (nutritional) value are also grouped under this category. Cigarettes, chewing gum, and candy are examples of this sort. These are probably not unconditioned reinforcers because there seems to be a history of learning or experience behind them. Generally speaking, certain stimuli or objects act as primary reinforcers because they have survival value. Obviously, some consumables do not have any such value.

Food as a primary reinforcer is used more often with certain populations than with other populations. Very young children, children who are nonverbal or minimally verbal, and persons who are profoundly retarded may often respond well to food as a reinforcer. Normally intelligent adults who seek clinical services may be so highly motivated to have their communicative disorders remediated that they react favorably to secondary reinforcers.

Food can be an effective reinforcer when used appropriately. Since its effects do not depend upon past learning or experience, clients who do not have much learning history behind them can be expected to be sensitive to food. This may be especially true of nonverbal or minimally verbal clients for whom words such as "good" and "excellent" may not mean much.

In many clinical studies, various articles of food have been used in training a variety of communicative behaviors. Cereal, ice cream, milk, candy, fruits, cookies, and other kinds of food have all been used in clinical sessions. In one of the early language training studies, for example, Guess, Sailor, Rutherford, and Baer (1968) used ice cream, Jello, mixed fruit, and milk as reinforcers while training mentally retarded children in the production of plural morphemes. Stevens-Long and Rasmussen (1974) also used food with autistic children who were being trained in the production of simple and compound sentence forms. Hegde and Gierut (1979) reinforced the correct production of several pronouns and a verb form ("are") in a four year old with candy and cereal. In teaching sign language to autistic children, Carr and Kologinsky (1983) gave small pieces of cheese as reinforcers. In each of these studies, the food items used were demonstrated to be reinforcers by documentation of systematic increases in the target behaviors under controlled conditions.

Limitations of Food as a Reinforcer. Although food can be a powerful reinforcer with some subjects, it has certain limitations. There are ways to overcome most of the limitations, and the clinician should be aware of them.

First, as a primary reinforcer, food can be effective only when it is deprived. In other words, a definite state of motivation must exist before food can act as a reinforcer. Therefore, it makes no sense to use cereal for reinforcers in a session conducted soon after the client had breakfast. If the child ate enough candy while taking the not too exciting ride to the speech clinic, candies may not act as reinforcers in the treatment sessions. The clinician must plan ahead when using food items as reinforcers. Most parents will cooperate if asked to withhold certain food items for several hours prior to the treatment sessions. Sessions can be so arranged that the food to be eaten for breakfast or lunch is actually eaten during clinical sessions held at appropriate times.

Second, food may not promote generalization and maintenance of communicative behaviors taught by the clinician. This is because food is not a natural reinforcer for speech and language behaviors. A majority of language response classes are more likely to be reinforced by conditioned (social) reinforcers. These are appropriate verbal and nonverbal responses from other people. Therefore, when food is used during training sessions, the language behaviors so learned may not easily generalize to other situations. This problem can be handled by simultaneous presentation of food and conditioned reinforcers. Eventually, food can be withdrawn in gradual steps while social reinforcers are still being used. This has been done in most of the clinical studies in which food was the reinforcer.

It must be noted, however, that there are some classes of verbal behaviors that typically receive primary reinforcers. These are called mands in behavioral analysis (Skinner, 1957; Winokur, 1976). Mands (commands, demands, requests) are made because of certain motivational states such as hunger or pain, and these are reinforced by the presentation of food or termination of the aversive event that caused the pain. For example, if the clinician were to train responses such as "can I have some juice please," the most appropriate reinforcer for this response would be some juice (primary reinforcer).

Third, food is very susceptible to the satiation effect. Even with appropriate levels of deprivation, the client may soon cease to work for food simply because of having had enough of it. This problem can be handled by the use of an intermittent reinforcement schedule in which food is given only for certain responses while certain other responses go unreinforced.

Fourth, food can create problems in presenting response contingently. Since dispensing food can be messy and time consuming, a delay between the response and the reinforcer may result. This is especially true in group therapy situations. It is difficult to reinforce correct responses given simultaneously by a group of clients (Kazdin, 1984).

Fifth, clients and parents may have certain objections to using foods or certain kinds of foods in clinical sessions. The clinician wishing to use food as a reinforcer should consult with the clients, parents, or both beforehand. In selecting food times, health related issues must be considered. When a client has problems such as diabetes and obesity, other kinds of reinforcers must be used.

Sixth, food can interrupt the sequence of training trials. If the child insists on eating every bit of cereal presented on each trial, the rate at which the training stimuli are presented can be retarded. The clinician would have to wait until the child chewed and swallowed the food before presenting the next trial. However, during the latter stages of treatment, children may be persuaded to save their reinforcers until the end of the session, or eat only some of them periodically.

Conditioned, or Social, Reinforcers

Social reinforcers are conditioned because their effects depend upon past learning. Phrases such as "fine job!" and "I like that" may not be reinforcing until a child has gone through certain experiences with them. Neutral stimuli acquire conditioned stimulus value because they may be associated with other reinforcing events. In caring for a young infant, the caregiver might smile, touch, and say nice words while feeding, bathing, holding, and playing with the child. Later on, the phrase "good job!" may suggest that a tangible reinforcer can be expected. Because of these reasons, certain neutral stimuli become reinforcers.

Social reinforcers are very appropriate in the treatment of communicative disorders. As suggested earlier, excluding mands, verbal behaviors are strengthened by social reinforcers. Therefore, it is natural to use them in teaching verbal responses. The most frequently used conditioned reinforcers include verbal praise, attention, touch, various facial expressions including smile, and eye contact. All of these can be powerful reinforcers with most individuals.

In many clinical studies, regardless of other reinforcers used, verbal reinforcers were always used. Hegde, Noll, and Pecora (1979), for example, used verbal reinforcers along with tokens in training a variety of grammatic features in two language delayed children. Campbell and Stremel-Campbell (1982) reinforced correct productions of three syntactic structures ("wh" questions, "yes-no" reversal questions, and statements) in two children, by using verbal praise. In making a comparative evaluation of oral and total communication programs with echolalic autistic children, Barrera and Sulzer-Azaroff (1983) paired social and edible reinforcers. In teaching a nonvocal communicaion system (Blissymbol versus iconic stimulus) to adolescents with severe physical disabilities, Hurlbut, Iwata, and Green (1982) also used verbal reinforcers such as "You're really working hard today" and "That's right!"

In the treatment of articulation disorders, verbal praise such as "good job," "excellent," and "I like that" has been used extensively (Elbert and McReynolds, 1975; Fitch, 1973; Bennett, 1974; Mowrer, 1977). For instance, Bailey, Timbers, Phillips, and Wolf (1971) showed that predelinquent youths' articulatory behaviors could be modified by training peers to administer verbal reinforcers for correct productions and punishers for incorrect ones. Bennett (1974) modified misarticulations of two hearing impaired girls with the verbal reinforcer "good!" Elbert and McReynolds (1975) also used verbal

"good!" as a reinforcer in training twelfth grade school children to produce /r/. In many studies, verbal reinforcers were combined with other
kinds of reinforcers such as tokens. Also, as noted earlier, wrong
responses were punished.

Social reinforcers are an integral part of many treatment programs in fluency disorders. Unfortunately, there are not many well
designed studies in which verbal reinforcers alone were shown to increase fluency. Nevertheless, treatment programs involving other
kinds of reinforcement contingencies generally use verbal reinforcers
as well. Many of the current treatment programs teach a stutterer to
slow down the speech rate, initiate speech sounds softly, prolong the
initial sound of words, and manage the airstream in certain ways to
produce and maintain fluent speech. In the treatment sessions, stutterers can be verbally reinforced for the production of such target
behaviors.

Conditioned reinforcers can be used just as well in treating voice
disorders, although once again there are not many well designed clinical studies. In treating various voice disorders, the clinician first identifies a target behavior such as a lower or higher pitch (compared with
the client's base rate), and shapes that target response in gradual
steps. Every time the client exhibits the target pitch level, the clinician verbally reinforces it.

In most clinical situations, multiple contingencies are used. For
example, verbal reinforcers may be paired with food or tokens. These
tokens may later be exchanged by the client for certain other kinds of
reinforcers. In addition, incorrect responses are typically punished by
verbal stimuli such as "wrong," timeout, or response cost. These and
other punishment procedures are described in Chapter 8.

Strengths and Weaknesses of Social Reinforcers. The
strengths of social reinforcers stem from the fact that they are conditioned reinforcers. First, they are not susceptible to satiation, as
primary reinforcers are. Apparently, people do not get easily tired of
verbal praise. Second, social reinforcers are more natural than the
primary, and for this reason may better promote generalization of
behaviors to extraclinical situations. Third, verbal stimuli such as
"good girl" and "excellent job" do not interrupt the sequence of target
behaviors. Fourth, when primary reinforcers must be used, the social
reinforcers can help fade them out. Initially, the two kinds of reinforcers can be paired with each other, and later, the primary reinforcer
can be withdrawn in gradual steps.

In spite of their strengths, social reinforcers may not always work.
As noted before, they tend to be least effective with clients who do
not have a history of verbal behavior. Profoundly retarded persons,

nonverbal clients, autistic children, and other persons lacking much experience with language may not initially react to smiles and verbal praise. In such cases, the clinician should establish the reinforcing value of social stimuli by systematically pairing them with primary reinforcers in the initial stages of training.

Conditioned Generalized Reinforcers

A class of very powerful reinforcers is known as conditioned generalized reinforcers. These reinforcers have been identified mostly through applied research with clinical populations exhibiting a variety of behavior disorders. Tokens, check marks on sheets of paper, marbles, stickers, points, and so on, can be conditioned generalized reinforcers, because once earned, they can be used to gain a variety of "true" reinforcers. Their effects do not depend upon a particular state of motivation. These reinforcers are powerful because their effects are generalized.

In everyday life, money is a conditioned generalized reinforcer. People work hard for it because it does what a generalized reinforcer does: it gives access to many other kinds of reinforcers. In the beginning, however, the conditioned generalized reinforcers may not be reinforcing by themselves. Their reinforcing value depends upon past experience. Eventually, they may be reinforcing in their own right, which is suggested by the fact that some people tend to hoard money.

In behavioral research, the effects of tokens have been researched extensively. Tokens were originally used in modifying behaviors of mental patients in institutions (Ayllon and Azrin, 1968). Since then, tokens have been used in a variety of clinical and educational settings in changing a wide range of behaviors. Several speech-language pathologists and audiologists have used tokens in their clinical work. The method has been used in modifying many aspects of communicative disorders.

At the outset of a token reinforcement program, tokens are simply given to the clients whose specific behavior is targeted for change. This is the initial noncontingent presentation of tokens. The clients are given a choice of backup reinforcers for which the tokens can be exchanged. Soon, the tokens are made to be response contingent. That is, the clients must perform the target behavior before tokens are presented. Studies have shown that this procedure can change behaviors rapidly (Kazdin, 1984).

Most frequently, plastic chips have been used as tokens. Check marks, stickers, points, marbles, and many other devices can be just as effective, however. All of these may be commonly referred to as tokens. A common mistake in using these devices is not to have a backup system of reinforcers. Some clinicians who claim to have used tokens may simply dispense marbles and plastic chips without backup reinforcers. Stickers given at the end of a session for being such a "good girl" or "good boy" may or may not be reinforcers.

Several studies illustrate the use of tokens in the treatment of articulation disorders. Johnston and Johnston (1972), for example, treated selected consonantal misarticulations in young children six to eight years of age. They were treated in small groups, and every time a child produced the target sounds correctly, a mark or dot or sticker was placed on that child's chart. A child who earned a certain number of these tokens could choose his or her favorite activity during the next free play period. The results showed a marked increase in the correct production of target consonants.

A study by Williams and McReynolds (1975) also illustrates the use of tokens in the treatment of articulation disorders. The study was designed to find out if auditory discrimination training was necessary to induce correct production of speech sounds. Four children, five to six years of age, were trained in individual sessions, and correct productions of target sounds were reinforced with marbles. During the sessions, the marbles were exchanged for plastic tokens, which were in turn exchanged for toys, candy, or both at the end of each session. The result of this study demonstrated the effectiveness of the token system in training correct articulation. Incidentally, auditory discrimination training did not increase production of target sounds, whereas production training did increase both production and discrimination.

In several language training studies, tokens were a part of the reinforcing contingency. In their study on language training, for example, Hegde, Noll, and Pecora (1979) presented a token (along with verbal reinforcers) for correct production of selected grammatic features. When ten tokens were accumulated, the child was allowed 2 minutes of play with a toy chosen at the beginning of the session. While training morphologic features in an adult mentally retarded female subject, Hegde and McConn (1981) reinforced correct responses with plastic tokens. As soon as ten tokens were accumulated, she was allowed to take a sip from a can of soda placed in front of her. With appropriate control procedures, both the studies demonstrated that the reinforcement contingency was effective.

A study by Jackson and Wallace (1974) illustrates the use of tokens in the treatment of voice disorders. A 15 year old aphonic girl received reinforcement with tokens for speaking with an intensity level required to operate a voice activated relay. If she did not speak with sufficient loudness, she would not activate the relay and thus would not get the token. With this procedure, the client was trained to speak with sufficient loudness in the clinical laboratory. However, additional shaping and reinforcement procedures were needed to have the treated vocal behavior generalized to extraclinical situations.

The effectiveness of tokens in the treatment of stuttering was evaluated in a series of studies by Ingham and his associates in Australia (see Ingham, 1984, for a review of these studies). In this treatment program, stutterers were hospitalized for as long as three weeks. The treatment involved delayed auditory feedback, which reduces the rate of speech and, presumably as a result, most forms of dysfluencies. The stutterers were required to earn tokens needed to purchase food, drink, and luxury items by exhibiting stutter-free speech in daily measurement sessions. The majority of stutterers were able to achieve stutter-free speech within the clinic when the token system was response contingent. The long-term effects in terms of generalization, maintenance, and speech quality either were not documented or were disappointing, however.

Clinicians who have used various recording symbols for measuring target behaviors may have noticed that different symbols used for correct and incorrect responses sometimes acquire reinforcing and punishing values. When a plus mark (+) has been used for correct responses that are reinforced, the child may begin to react to it the way he or she would to the actual reinforcer. Similarly, the child may react to minus signs (−) that may have been associated with punished responses as though they were punishing stimuli, even in the absence of the actual punishing consequence. These observations are suggestive of the way the conditioned reinforcers develop.

Strengths and Weaknessess of Conditioned Generalized Reinforcers. Conditioned generalized reinforcers have several advantages. First, their effects do not depend upon a single state of deprivation. Because tokens or points can be exchanged for a variety of reinforcers, it can be assumed that at any given time the client would "work for" one or the other of those backups. Therefore, conditioned generalized reinforcers are not susceptible to satiation effects.

Second, tokens and points are easy to administer to either individuals or groups. When they are administered to a group, different individuals can receive different backup reinforcers. Third, tokens can be administered without interrupting the sequence of target behaviors. There is no time loss due to consumption of food even when food is used as a backup reinforcer. Fourth, tokens can be very useful when a particular reinforcer selected by a client is judged very valuable, and therefore the contingency requires a lot of work. For example, if a visit to the campus library is a backup reinforcer, the clinician can let the child accumulate the necessary number of tokens or points. In this way, a large reinforcer can be earned in stages by cumulative work.

The limitations of a token system are mostly practical. First, the clinician should have a variety of backup reinforcers available all the time. If not, there is no particular advantage in using a token system. An effective backup system can be expensive to maintain. Second, when tokens are withdrawn, sometimes a sudden decline in behaviors may be seen (Kazdin, 1984), although this problem is not unique to tokens. Any system of reinforcement should be withdrawn in gradual steps. Whenever tokens are given, social reinforcers can and should be administered also, so that the behaviors can be maintained by the latter.

Informative Feedback

Informative feedback is a form of conditioned reinforcer, but it deserves special consideration because of its unique nature. During treatment, many clients find it reinforcing to know where they stand in relation to a criterion of performance set by the clinician. Informative feedback provides such specific information to the client. Although informative feedback is often very similar to verbal reinforcers, there are at least two important distinctions. First, feedback need not be verbal at all, as in the case of biofeedback. Mechanical feedback of information regarding a client's performance can be just as reinforcing. Second, even when verbal feedback is given, it need not be in the form of praise. It can be an objective statement regarding the level of performance in relation to a previously specified target criterion. Of course, informative feedback can be combined with verbal praise, other kinds of reinforcers, or both.

The number of clinical experiments in which informative feedback has been used in treating communicative disorders is relatively small. Most of these studies have been done in the areas of voice and fluency. Some very early experiments in the modification of voice disorders with the help of mechanical feedback were done by Roll in the late 1960s. These unpublished studies are cited in Fitch (1973). Essentially, Roll was able to show that with the help of mechanical filters, it is possible to isolate a target vocal fundamental frequency in clients with pitch disorders. Using electronic relay systems, he was able to reinforce target pitch levels with informative feedback.

Another study by Roll (1973) was concerned with hypernasality in children with cleft palate. One subject's cleft palate was surgically repaired, but there was still a mild hypernasality. The other subject had a cleft of the soft palate and severe hypernasality. The treatment consisted of a mechanical feedback in the form of a white light for nonnasal productions of (nonnasal) speech sounds, and a red light for nasal productions. No other reinforcers were given. The subjects were simply told to "make the white light come on" every time a speech sound was produced. This type of differential visual feedback was shown to be effective in reducing undesirable nasal resonance in speech. A withdrawal design was used to demonstrate the experimental control over nasality.

One of the most extensively researched aspects of informative feedback is known as biofeedback. In biofeedback, the clinician gives information regarding the client's various physiological functions, such as blood pressure and heart rate, with the help of mechanical devices. For example, in the treatment of stuttering, various muscle activities measured by electromyography (EMG), electrical conductance of the skin measured by galvanic skin response (GSR), and electrical activity of the cerebral cortex measured by electroencephalography (EEG) have been investigated (Ingham, 1984). Of these, EMG has been monitored most frequently, presumably because stuttering seems to be associated with some degree of tension in speech related muscles.

Procedurally, the physiological function of interest is measured and displayed in either visual or auditory form. The client is instructed to maintain the display or change it in some manner. For example, the stutterer might be asked to reduce the level of muscle activity from the basal level in gradual steps. As the activity level decreases, the display changes, providing immediate feedback to the client.

By and large, feedback-based procedures have not proved to be very effective in the treatment of stuttering. Clinical studies done so far have had methodological problems. Therefore, it is not clear whether poor results were due to faulty studies or to some inherent weakness in informative feedback itself. Some recent developments in the treatment of stuttering suggest the possibility that feedback procedures may be more effective in treating stuttering if the target is certain phonatory behaviors. It is known that when stutterers increase their voicing durations or prolong the initial sounds of words, they tend to be less dysfluent. Recently, mechanical feedback of voicing durations has been shown to be a potential treatment technique (Ingham, Montgomery, and Ulliana, 1983).

Strengths and Weaknesses of Informative Feedback. There is not much valid, replicated data in the field of communicative disorders to evaluate the eventual usefulness of feedback procedures. This is especially true of mechanical feedback of information regarding physiological activity in clients with speech and language disorders. Available information is somewhat sketchy and disappointing. Verbal feedback, on the other hand, is almost always a part of contingencies involving other kinds of reinforcers. When a clinician sets a performance criterion for the client, and reinforces verbally, information regarding the performance will have been given to the client automatically. Eventually, any kind of reinforcer will come to give such feedback to the client. This might suggest that pure feedback regarding performance levels may be less effective than the feedback inherent in other kinds of reinforcers.

Informative feedback, including biofeedback, has been extensively tested in the treatment of behavioral disorders, including headaches, hypertension, anxiety and phobic reactions, cardiac arrhythmias, epileptic seizures, and so on. Even there, questions have always been raised about the durability of pure feedback effects (Kazdin, 1984). At the present, mechanical use of feedback procedures must be considered experimental in communicative disorders. Treatment of voice disorders and treatment of stuttering based on phonatory modifications probably hold the greatest promise.

High Probability Behaviors

So far, things and events that are reinforcing have been described. When a response is made, some object or a stimulus is presented to the person exhibiting that response. It may be a spoonful of cereal, a verbal stimulus such as "good!", a token, a check mark, or informative feedback. A reinforcer, however, need not be a stimulus or a thing presented by someone else. It can be an opportunity to engage in some type of activity. The reinforcer in this case is the client's own behavior. Obviously, this behavior is something other than the target behavior the clinician is trying to establish. This type of reinforcer was originally described by a behavioral scientist named Premack. Therefore, the underlying principle is sometimes described as the Premack principle.

The Premack principle states that a behavior of high probability can reinforce a behavior of low probability. It is important to note that both the response to be reinforced and the reinforcer are behaviors of the same person. The clinician in this situation controls the opportunities for the high probability behaviors, which are made contingent upon the low probability behaviors.

The clinical targets, by definition, are low probability behaviors. Whether it is the correct productions of certain speech sounds, morphologic features, or elements of a manual sign language, the target behaviors are not exhibited at high probability. If they were, there would be no need for any special services. At the same time, the children and adults who seek help are also capable of certain behaviors that they may be exhibiting at very high frequency. If these behaviors can be made contingent upon clinical targets, then a potential reinforcer will have been found.

The Premack principle is operative in everyday life. Whenever possible, people control access to desirable behaviors so that certain least preferred actions are performed first. Parents know that watching television is a high probability behavior in the case of most children. At the same time, homework may be a low probability behavior. A majority of children are not likely to engage in solving math problems or reading history textbooks on their own. If parents wish to increase such academic behaviors, they can then make the television watching contingent upon finishing certain homework. Similarly, parents might ask the child to eat vegetables before eating meat. An adult might mow the lawn before watching a football game on television.

In order to find out the high probability behaviors, the clinician must observe the client in an unrestrained situation to see the "natural" and relative frequencies of several behaviors. If one of these behaviors is exhibited very consistently and at a high rate, and if opportunities for that behavior can be controlled by the clinician, then the Premack principle can be used in therapy. Typically, information gathered from the family members of a client can be useful in selecting potential high probability behaviors.

There are not many controlled studies in which the effectiveness of the Premack principle in the treatment of communicative disorders has been specifically evaluated. There are some clinical studies in which high probability behaviors were used as backup reinforcers for tokens. They illustrate the Premack principle all the same.

The children who earned tokens for correct productions of speech sounds in the previously quoted Johnston and Johnston (1972) study were allowed to choose an activity during the following play time. In the study by Hegde, Noll, and Pecora (1979), one of the children under language training was given tokens that were exchanged for 2 minutes of play. In both the studies, the high probability play activity served as a reinforcer for the low probability speech or language behaviors that were being trained.

Various activities that children exhibit very frequently can be programmed to act as reinforcers. Clinicians know that activities such as looking into comic books or pictures, reading story books, various leisure time activities, listening to music, coloring and other art-related activities, playing with specific toys, imaginary games played with other children are typically high probability behaviors in most children. These activities are potential reinforcers of target behaviors in clinical sessions.

A word of caution in the use of high probability behaviors is in order. Some speech and language pathologists may use "free play" as a form of treatment. Often, such "free play" is simply an uncontrolled and noncontingent activity that may not reinforce anything. From a treatment standpoint, it may be a waste of time. There is a difference between "free play" and play activity as a response-contingent event whose effect upon that response is constantly measured to make sure that it is a reinforcer.

A clinician who wishes to use a high probability behavior for a reinforcer must make sure that it is made contingent upon the clinical target behaviors. In other words, the client should earn those activities by exhibiting the target behaviors. In most individual therapy sessions, high probability behaviors are parceled out depending upon the number of correct responses produced by the client. Tokens and check marks are useful in administering high probability behaviors response contingently.

Strengths and Weaknesses of High Probability Behaviors. With most clients, it is possible to identify very strong response trends. Once established, high probability behaviors can be very effective reinforcers as long as they are made response contingent. In many cases, they may be more effective than primary or social reinforcers. When the treatment sessions are long, brief breaks during which earned activity is permitted can help reduce the monotony. Often, different high probability behaviors can be identified for a given client so that there is a "pool of reinforcers" constantly available to the clinician.

The weaknesses of the high probability concept of reinforcement are mostly practical. First, it is often not possible to make the high probability behavior contingent upon target behaviors. An opportunity to play for a few minutes, for example, cannot be made available for every correct production of a target phoneme or grammatic morpheme. Second, as reinforcers, high probability behaviors are perhaps the most time consuming. Therefore, high probability behaviors cannot be used during the initial stages of training when every response must be reinforced. A solution to these two problems is to give tokens for correct responses and have high probability behaviors as backup reinforcers. In this way, a child would still be reinforced for every correct response with tokens, and the play activity would be available when a certain number of tokens have been accumulated.

Third, some of the high probability behaviors are presented either in total or not at all (Kazdin, 1984). If the child must earn 25 tokens in order to be able to listen to music at the end of the session, and if the number of tokens actually earned falls short of the criterion, then the child may have to go totally unreinforced. To avoid this situation, a very low criterion of correct responses may be required in the beginning. This criterion may be raised in gradual steps as the client's response rate improves. Backup reinforcers are made available to the client in each step of the treatment.

MULTIPLE CONTINGENCIES

So far, a variety of positive reinforcers have been considered that can be used in treating communicative disorders. It is the responsibility of the clinician to select an event that is reinforcing to a given client. The events just described are not expected to actually act as reinforcers for all clients, for all behaviors, and across time. The technical definition of a reinforcer should always be kept in perspective. In training a particular response at a given time, an empirical reinforcer can be determined by repeatedly measuring the response rate.

In most treatment sessions, it is desirable to use multiple contingencies. Verbal reinforcers are almost always used along with primary reinforcers. Verbal reinforcers may be combined with tokens backed up by high probability behaviors. In addition to positive reinforcers, the clinician may often find it necessary to use punishing contingencies to decrease certain interfering and undesirable behaviors. In most treatment sessions, the clinician will concurrently manage multiple reinforcing and punishing contingencies.

NEGATIVE REINFORCERS

So far, positive reinforcers that increase response rates have been discussed. The second major category of events that increases response rates is known as negative reinforcers. In the positive reinforcement procedure, an event or a stimulus is presented response contingently. In the negative reinforcement procedure, events or stimuli are removed response contingently. The events that are removed are often described as aversive. When aversive events are removed or terminated response contingently, then those responses tend to increase in frequency. Such an increase defines the negative reinforcement procedure.

Negative reinforcement should not be confused with punishment. In punishment, response rates decrease, whereas in negative reinforcement, the rates increase. These two are opposite processes with contrasting effects on response rates. Unfortunately, some clinicians use the term negative reinforcement when they actually mean punishment. It is important to note that both positive and negative reinforcement procedures have the same effect on the response rates, while the punishment has the opposite effect.

Everyone knows that people tend to move away from events, stimuli, and people that are aversive. Some aversive stimuli, such as excessive heat, cold, or noise, may cause physical harm. Some aversive events have negative effects that may not be immediate but delayed. Rooms filled with cigarette smoke, for example, are immediately aversive, but their physical effects may be delayed.

Some events or stimuli may not have any undesirable physical effects but may still be aversive enough so people would prefer not to experience them. A boring person, telephone calls from sales persons, screaming children, noisy neighbors, and excessive talkers are some of the stimuli that people tend to move away from. When people are confronted with such events, they tend to do something that would terminate those events. Those actions that are successful in terminating specific aversive events tend to be repeated. For example, if a parent tells the screaming children to go to their room, and the children obey, the aversive screaming will have been terminated. As a result, and in the future, the parent is more likely to tell the children to go to their room whenever they are noisy. It can then be said that the parent's response of asking the children to go to their room has been negatively reinforced. The frequency of the parent's request increased because it was successful in terminating the aversive, noisy behavior on the part of the children.

Escape and Avoidance

Research on learning and conditioning has suggested that two types of behaviors are generated by aversive events. The first type is called escape, and the second type is called avoidance. In escape, the person actually comes in contact with the aversive event and does something to terminate it. In avoidance, on the other hand, the person does something so that the aversive event is not experienced at all. Generally speaking, first there is escape, and soon there is avoidance.

If a person who invites himself to your table at a cafeteria starts to ruin a pleasant lunch hour, you and your friends may finish your lunch in a hurry and get out of that place. This is escape behavior, since you did come in contact with the aversive person. On the other hand, if you find out that this person regularly eats lunch at a certain time, you may decide to go to lunch earlier or later, so that you simply do not come into contact with that person. As an extreme response, you may even start eating lunch at a different restaurant. These are avoidance behaviors. You escape from an aversive situation you are already in, and avoid the one you expect to get into. In either case, the behavior is reinforced negatively. The process of teaching new behaviors or increasing the frequency of existing behaviors through negative reinforcement is called avoidance conditioning.

It is obvious that in the example just given, escape behavior came before the avoidance behavior. But one can learn to avoid a situation without first having escaped from it. In human behavior, this often happens because of the benefit of the verbal contingency. Your friend tells you not to go to a certain part of the town because it is dangerous, and you don't, even though you have never seen that part of the town. This is avoidance without prior escape. When people follow safety rules, various kinds of verbal advice, and so on, they are avoiding consequences of certain behaviors without having exhibited those behaviors.

Escape and avoidance behaviors and the ensuing negative reinforcement have been extensively studied in animal research, but have been used only occasionally in the treatment of behavior disorders. Aversive stimuli such as loud noise and electric shock have been used to modify some problem behaviors within an aversive conditioning paradigm. One of the reasons why avoidance conditioning has not been used very frequently in clinical treatment is that positive reinforcement is preferable to negative reinforcement. Because both are capable of increasing response rates, one may as well use the positive reinforcement procedure. Some clinicians believe that aversive techniques may have certain undesirable side effects of the kind noted with punishment procedures (see Chapter 8).

In the treatment of communicative disorders, there are not many examples of negative reinforcement. In order to use it as a treatment procedure, an aversive stimulus must be presented continuously. The stimulus is terminated whenever a desirable response is given by the client. In this manner, the desirable response is reinforced negatively.

The literature on the experimental analysis of stuttering contains a few examples of negative reinforcement. In fact, one of the earliest studies on the operant conditioning of stuttering, done by Flanagan,

Goldiamond, and Azrin (1958) involved negative reinforcement as well as punishment. In the negative reinforcement portion of the study, an aversive noise of 6,000 Hz was continuously presented through earphones at 105 dB. Every time the subject stuttered, however, the noise was turned off for 5 seconds. The authors reported an increase in stuttering as a result of this negative reinforcement. In the punishment condition, the noise was made contingent upon stuttering, resulting in a decrease in stuttering rate. Both the contingencies were removed in subsequent conditions of the study, thus returning the rate of stuttering to its usual level. Obviously, the authors' purpose was to demonstrate that stuttering was an operant behavior that could be increased or decreased by arranging certain consequences. The negative reinforcement portion of the study was not intended to suggest a potential treatment for stuttering. It was fully expected to increase the rate of stuttering.

The need to provide a constant aversive stimulus before it can be terminated response contingently makes the negative reinforcement procedure less attractive for clinical purposes. Aversive stimuli are more frequently used in decreasing undesirable responses than in increasing desirable behaviors. This means that aversive events may be better used as punishment and not as (negative) reinforcement.

Summary. Techniques designed to increase target behaviors during clinical training have been discussed. The two major techniques that increase behaviors are positive and negative reinforcement. The following five types of positive reinforcers were also discussed: primary reinforcers, secondary reinforcers, conditioned generalized reinforcers, informative feedback, and high probability behaviors. All types of positive reinforcement are achieved through response contingent presentation of a stimulus, whereas negative reinforcement is achieved by the termination of an ongoing aversive event. Both the procedures increase response rates. Theoretically, it is possible to use negative reinforcement clinically, but not many reports describe the application of this procedure in increasing communicative behaviors.

SCHEDULES OF REINFORCEMENT

A reinforcing consequence can be given for every correct response or only for some of them. Early laboratory research on response consequences has produced a wealth of information on what came to be known as the schedules of reinforcement (Ferster and

Skinner, 1957). In this section, the major schedules that have been used in clinical treatment will be summarized.

A schedule of reinforcement can be defined as a relation between (1) the number of responses and the amount of reinforcement, or (2) responses and the time duration between the delivery of reinforcers. To put it simply, schedules specify how many responses will be required before a reinforcer is given or when it will be given. The reinforcement schedules used during training will determine to some extent whether the response will be acquired relatively slowly or quickly, whether it will be maintained or extinguished as soon as the reinforcer is withdrawn, and whether the response will have a potential for generalization or not. Needless to say, these are important treatment considerations.

There are two broad categories of reinforcement schedules: continuous and intermittent. Furthermore, there are several types of intermittent schedules. Each schedule has its strengths and weaknesses and generates a distinct pattern of responses. The major schedules, their characteristic effects on response rates, and their clinical use will be described.

Continuous Reinforcement

In the continuous reinforcement schedule, every response is reinforced. In clinical situations, however, every response means every correct response. In the early stages of treatment, clients are more likely to give both correct and incorrect responses. Only the target correct responses are reinforced by the clinician, and incorrect responses are punished or extinguished (ignored). In clinical practice, then, the continuous reinforcement is interrupted by a continuous punishment schedule administered for incorrect responses.

Social reinforcers can be very easily administered on a continuous basis. Some other reinforcers, such as high probability behaviors, are not efficiently administered continuously. However, as noted earlier, when high probability behaviors are used as backup reinforcers, tokens or check marks can be delivered on a continuous basis.

A major strength of continuous reinforcement is that it can help generate a very high rate of response. When a response is either totally absent or present only at a very low level of frequency, continuous reinforcement can be very useful in shaping that response or increasing its frequency. However, continuous reinforcement has a distinct weakness that the clinician must be aware of. Behaviors generated and shaped by continuous reinforcement may not be sustained when that kind of reinforcement is no longer available. Withholding reinforcers for a response is known as extinction and the procedure typically results in a decreased rate of response. Continuously reinforced responses are highly susceptible to extinction.

Intermittent Schedules of Reinforcement

There are several schedules in which reinforcers are delivered intermittently. Four schedules that have clinical applications to varying degrees will be described. Two of these are dependent upon the number of responses; the other two are dependent upon the time interval between reinforcers. The former are called ratio schedules with two variations: fixed ratio and variable ratio. The latter are called interval schedules, also with two variations: fixed interval and variable interval.

Fixed Ratio Schedules. Under a fixed ratio schedule, a predetermined number of responses is required before a reinforcer is delivered. For example, in the treatment of an articulation disorder, a clinician might reinforce every fifth correct response. This would then be a fixed ratio of five. The schedule is often abbreviated FR, followed by a number that specifies how many responses are required for reinforcement. An FR2 would mean that every second response is reinforced, and an FR50 would mean that every 50th response is reinforced.

Laboratory studies have shown that responses generated by fixed ratio schedules have certain important characteristics. First, between reinforcers, the response rate is very high. Once the initial response is made, the ratio requirement is completed rapidly. For example, under an FR20 schedule, as soon as the first response (after the last reinforcement) is made, the remaining 19 responses are made with very little hesitation in between responses. Second, reinforcement typically results in a distinct pause in the response rate. The subject tends to "rest" a little after every time the ratio requirement is completed and the reinforcer is received. This rest period is known as the postreinforcement pause. Third, the length of the postreinforcement pause is determined by the size of the ratio. The larger the ratio, the greater the duration of pauses.

The three characteristics of the fixed ratio schedule results in an "all or none" pattern of responses. The person is either working very hard, or resting. There are not many periods of lazy, slow, and unsure responding. High response rates and rest periods constitute a cyclical pattern under fixed ratios. Arrangements in many work-related situations approximate fixed ratio schedules. In agriculture, seasonal workers are typically paid on the basis of the number of bushels, boxes, or baskets that the workers fill with picked cotton, fruit, or vegetables. In the garment industry, payment may be contingent upon a certain number of dresses sewn. This type of arrangement, known as "piecework," is similar to fixed ratio schedules and can generate a very high production rate.

Ratio schedules can not only generate high response rates but also make people work harder while receiving progressively less and less reinforcement. Laboratory studies have shown that if the ratio is stretched in small and gradual steps, response rates can be maintained on very large ratios that deliver minimum reinforcement. Pigeons' pecking responses, for example, have been maintained on FR20,000. The history of industrial production shows that in some cases people have been made to work harder and harder while being paid less and less.

When the ratio must be increased, it must be done in gradual steps. An FR2 may be initially increased to an FR4, but perhaps not to FR20. Large, abrupt shifts result in prolonged periods of no reinforcement resulting in response extinction. This is often described as a ratio strain.

In several clinical studies, different fixed ratios of reinforcement have been used. Generally speaking, very large ratios have not been used, presumably because the clients needed lower ratios. Fixed ratios of 2, 3, or 4 have been used frequently. However, when tokens are used, a large number of correct responses can be required before they are exchanged for backup reinforcers. In the Hegde, Noll, and Pecora (1979) study on language training, for example, ten tokens were required before the child could engage in 2 minutes of play activity.

Variable Ratio Schedules. A reinforcement schedule more powerful than the fixed ratio is known as the variable ratio (VR). Under this schedule, the number of responses required for reinforcement keeps varying from occasion to occasion. However, such variations are not random. They are based on an average number of responses. A VR20, for example, would suggest that on the average 20 responses are made before reinforcement, but from time to time, the actual number of responses needed to receive the reinforcer is varied around 20. Sometimes the reinforcer is given just after one or two responses, but at other times many more responses are required. Under a specific variable ratio schedule, there is typically an upper limit on the number of responses required for reinforcement.

Theoretically, persons responding under a variable ratio schedule cannot discriminate when the reinforcer is actually going to be delivered. It might appear that every response has an equal chance of being reinforced. The fact that the previous response was reinforced may not mean that the next one will not be reinforced. Presumably because of such a lack of discrimination, persons tend to respond more consistently under the variable ratio than under the fixed ratio.

Several specific characteristics of the response rates generated by variable ratio schedules have been identified. First, response rates under variable ratio schedules are typically high. Second, there is no marked postreinforcement pause under the variable schedule. Third, a high response rate is more steady and consistent under the variable than under the fixed ratio.

A lack of postreinforcement pause is probably responsible for a steadier response rate under a variable ratio. In fixed ratios, the delivery of a reinforcer means that the next or the next several responses will not be reinforced, resulting in a pause in responding. Under variable schedules, on the other hand, consecutive responses may be reinforced on occasions, and therefore the subject does not pause soon after receiving a reinforcer.

It is quite possible that in everyday situations, reinforcers are more likely to come on a variable basis than on a fixed ratio. For instance, you may not find an interesting letter every time you check the mail box. Nor would you consistently find it on every fifth or fiftieth try. Thus, the mail box checking behavior is not reinforced either continuously or on a fixed ratio basis. You may find something interesting every day for a few consecutive days, and then several days of junk mail in quantity may follow. Then suddenly, a long-awaited tax refund may show up. This kind of variable schedule produces a very strong response rate that resists extinction. Days and days of junk mail or even no mail will not deter most people from checking the box regularly.

It is thought that the persistence of gambling and such other undesirable behaviors may be due to the influence of variable ratios of reinforcement. A person playing at a slot machine is often unable to predict the occurrence of a payoff. Any pull on the handle might make the person rich, or so it seems to the compulsive gambler. This is thought to be a result of the indiscriminable nature of variable ratios.

In controlled clinical studies, variable ratios have been used somewhat less frequently than the fixed ratios. Administration of a variable schedule takes more planning than does a fixed schedule. In laboratory studies, electronic programming devices vary the number of responses from occasion to occasion while still maintaining a fixed average. As long as the device receives response inputs (such as a bar press), the reinforcer may be delivered automatically.

In routine clinical situations, variable schedules are often administered more informally. Within a narrow range, a different number of responses may be required on different occasions of reinforcement. For example, at a certain stage in the treatment of an articulation disorder, four to seven correct responses may be required before the reinforcer is made available. At any given time, a specific number of responses would be required, but it would vary across reinforcement opportunities. If the range of variations is relatively small, the clinician can execute a variable schedule efficiently without sophisticated programming equipment.

A study involving five deaf children illustrates the effectiveness of variable ratio schedules in a special classroom setting (Van Houten and Nau, 1980). The authors compared the effects of VR8 and VR12 with FR8 and FR12 schedules. The study revealed that the deaf children's visual attending behaviors were better during the VR conditions than during the FR conditions. The children were also able to solve more math problems under the VR schedules than under the FR schedules.

A language training study cited earlier illustrates the use of a VR3. Campbell and Stremel-Campbell (1982) trained two retarded children in the correct production of certain questions and statements. In the training phase, the children's correct productions of target behaviors were continuously reinforced with verbal praise and tokens. After a given target reached the training criterion, a maintenance phase was introduced. In this phase, productions of question forms or statements were reinforced on a VR3. The authors used a "loose training" strategy (described in Chapter 9) and showed that the procedures were effective in obtaining a generalized production of the target behaviors.

Just like larger fixed ratios, variable ratio schedules can also be very useful in fading the reinforcer programmed during the initial stages of training. With proper planning, the ratio can be increased in gradual steps, thus making it difficult for the client to discriminate the occasions of reinforcement from those of no reinforcement. Once again, this schedule might better approximate the natural environment and promote response generalization and maintenance.

In ratio schedules the critical variable is the number of responses made by the subject. In interval schedules, on the other hand, what is critical is a time duration between reinforcers. For this reason, these schedules are sometimes described as time dependent. Two basic time dependent schedules will be described: fixed interval and variable interval.

Fixed Interval Schedules. In a fixed interval schedule, an opportunity to earn a reinforcer is made available after the passage of a fixed duration of time. The very first response made after the interval is over is reinforced. It must be noted that although time dependent schedules specify a certain fixed or average duration, they also require a response before a reinforcer can be obtained. The fixed duration may be over, but if the specified response is not made, the reinforcer will not be forthcoming. That is why the schedule is defined in terms of an opportunity to earn a reinforcer by responding soon after the duration is over. The interval of time measured is typically the duration between reinforcers.

The fixed interval schedule is abbreviated FI, and an FI5-minutes means that the reinforcer is delivered for the first response made 5 minutes after the previous reinforced response. Laboratory studies have shown that FI schedules have effects that are somewhat similar to the FR schedules. However, overall response rates under FI schedules can be lower (less consistent) than those under FR schedules. This is probably because responses made within the interval are not reinforced, and therefore not many responses are made soon after a reinforcer has been received. Indeed, there is usually a very distinct pause in the response rate following the delivery of a reinforcer. The pause durations are often longer than those found under the FR schedules. The actual durations are a function of the fixed interval. The longer the interval, the greater the pause duration after the reinforcement.

Another characteristic of FI schedules is that responses increase gradually as the time passes, and they reach their highest rate just before the interval is about to end. Thus, the typical response rates under FI schedules show a pattern of concentrated responses around the interval, a distinct pause after the reinforcer has been given, and a slow pickup of the response rate.

Although strict fixed interval schedules are not so common in everyday situations, many behaviors are probably maintained by similar types of contingencies. Suppose you are expecting a letter with a job offer in the mail, and you can see the mailperson's vehicle through your window. Assuming that your mail typically is delivered around 12 noon, you probably begin to glance down the street several minutes before that time. Initially, these glances will be occasional. Soon, however, they become more and more frequent, and at or around 12 noon, you are constantly looking out into the street in the hope of spotting the mailperson. Soon after the delivery of mail (regardless of whether you received the expected letter or not), you are not likely to look out for the mailperson again until around noon time the next day. This response pattern approximates the characteristics of behaviors generated and maintained by fixed interval schedules.

Another everyday example of behaviors that approximate the effects of fixed interval reinforcement can be found in the study habits of college students. When, at the beginning of a semester, an instructor assigns a term paper due in six weeks, you are not likely to rush home and burn the midnight oil. You probably will not give much thought to it during the initial week or two. Then you begin to hear the unsettling story that some of your friends have already done some work on their papers while you were having a good time. You begin to put some time into your paper. Initially, you may spend only a few minutes reading or thinking about it. But as the inevitable due date comes closer, you start spending more and more time on the paper. Finally, the day before the due date, you may be missing from parties, bars, beaches, and all classes as well. Everyone knows what you are doing at this time. When the paper is finished and turned in, you may not rush to the library to do some reading on a project due in four weeks. You probably head toward a more interesting place for an "I deserve it" type of experience.

Fixed interval schedules have not been used in applied research as frequently as fixed ratio schedules. In clinical treatment sessions, fixed interval schedules may not be as efficient as fixed ratio schedules, because the objective is to evoke responses continuously during the session. An interval schedule generates concentrated responses mostly around the time when the specified duration is about to expire. It does not encourage responses during the interval, which may lead to an inefficient use of treatment time available during sessions.

In the treatment of voice and fluency disorders, what appears to be a fixed interval schedule may sometimes be used. For example, the clinician may require a client to speak with a certain pitch, or maintain fluency for a certain duration of time. The client may be reinforced for such time-based responses (Hegde and Brutten, 1978). But these are not strictly fixed interval schedules, since clients are required to maintain target behaviors throughout the specified time interval.

Variable Interval Schedules. When the time interval between reinforcers is allowed to vary from time to time, we have the variable interval schedule (VI). In this arrangement, the required intervals between reinforcers are varied around an average. A VI5-minutes means that on the average, the first response made 5-minutes after the last reinforcement is reinforced. Across occasions, however, the duration of actual intervals will be different. Sometimes the required duration may be more than 5-minutes; at other times it may be less. But the variations are arranged in such a way that the average duration between reinforcers is 5-minutes. Just as in the fixed interval schedule, the passage of time alone will not result in the delivery of a reinforcer. The person must give the specified response in order to receive the reinforcer.

Experimental research has shown that variable interval schedules generate a steady (consistent) response rate. Because of this consistency, the overall rate tends to be higher under variable than under fixed interval schedules. The number of responses may be high or low depending upon the specific duration of the interval. The shorter the duration, the higher the response rate, and vice versa. The schedule does not generate distinct postreinforcement pauses. Instead, it shapes a persistent and evenly spaced response rate, which may be somewhat lower than that found under variable ratio schedules. It is thought that those who work hard consistently, but are not especially fast, may have been exposed to variable interval schedules of reinforcement.

Probably many of our everyday behaviors are shaped by schedules that are similar to variable interval schedules. Supervisors who check on workers at variable times may encourage more consistent work than those who check at regular intervals. When students are taking an examination, the instructor may walk around the class to make sure that no one is cheating. If the instructor keeps changing the "route" so that he or she ends up checking each student at varying intervals, the students will be working under a schedule similar to variable interval schedules.

Application of the variable interval schedule in the modification of communicative behaviors has been very limited. By and large, clinicians have tried to modify behaviors by actually controlling the number of responses more directly. Ratio schedules permit a more direct manipulation of the number of responses the clients exhibit. Also, the clinical treatment sessions are usually limited in time. Therefore, it becomes difficult to effectively arrange varying time schedules. Under gradually increasing ratio schedules, clients have to give more and more responses, and clinicians appropriately tend to capitalize on this tendency.

Differential Reinforcement of Other Behaviors. A special type of reinforcement schedule that has been used in clinical settings is known as the differential reinforcement of other behavior (DRO).

Most schedules specify what specific responses and how many responses will be reinforced. In a DRO, on the other hand, what is specified is a behavior that will not be reinforced.

In clinical situations, clients often exhibit certain unwanted behaviors such as leaving the chair, crying, or looking away from the clinician. A given child may have a specific noncooperative behavior (say chewing on the shirt collar) during the treatment sessions. Under the DRO schedule, the clinician would reinforce the child as long as the collar chewing behavior is not exhibited. What desirable behaviors must be exhibited may not be specified. A variety of responses, including looking at the pictures, sitting in a certain posture, responding to clinicians's modeling, and many others, may be reinforced. The essential feature of the schedule is that behaviors to be reinforced may be many, varied, and left unspecified, whereas what will not be reinforced is clearly specified.

Many clinicians probably routinely use the DRO schedule in controlling uncooperative behaviors by reinforcing a variety of cooperative behaviors. Possibly, the schedule is used more frequently with young children. Whenever the clinician tells the child that "if you don't do this, you will get this" (and follows through with expected results), the DRO schedule may be involved. A child may be given a token for not yawning during ten training trials. Another child may be reinforced for not wiggling in the chair during the previous few minutes. Yet another child may be reinforced for not looking into the observational mirror while the clinician is trying to have the attention focused upon a stimulus picture. While the child is not doing this or that specified action, any number or variety of other behaviors may be reinforced.

In the treatment of stuttering, the clinician may specify behaviors that are considered stutterings, and tell clients that as long as they continue to speak without those behaviors, reinforcement can be expected. It is possible that many of the currently effective stuttering treatment programs make use of this schedule of reinforcement. Most clinicians try to establish a pattern of speech that is devoid of specified stuttering behaviors. Initially, this pattern of speech may be slow and prolonged, and thus not really the final target behavior. Nevertheless, this new pattern of speech may be reinforced because it does not contain behaviors considered stutterings. Once a nonstuttering speech pattern has been learned to a certain extent, that pattern may be changed by shaping the normal rate, prosody, or other features. In this phase of treatment, the initially learned, slow, prolonged pattern may itself become the behavior that would not be reinforced. In order to earn reinforcers, the client would then have to speak with normal rate and prosody while still not exhibiting stuttering behaviors.

Similar strategies can be used in the treatment of voice disorders. A client with an undesirable pitch may be reinforced as long as that particular pitch level is not exhibited while he or she is saying words or sentences. Assuming that the new pitch is in the direction of the final target, it may be reinforced simply because it is not the undesirable baseline pitch of the client. Once again, the schedule is the DRO.

The DRO has a tremendous potential in controlling undesirable behaviors by increasing the desirable ones. It must be noted that although the schedule may have an indirect effect of decreasing certain behaviors, it does so by increasing incompatible behaviors. Hence, the schedule involves a positive reinforcement contingency and therefore should not be confused with punishment.

CLINICAL USE OF DIFFERENT REINFORCEMENT SCHEDULES

The strengths and weaknesses of different reinforcement schedules have important clinical implications. The clinician is initially concerned with either shaping a new behavior or increasing the frequency of an existing behavior. The clinician is also concerned with generalization and maintenance of newly shaped or increased behaviors. Unfortunately, what is best for the initial training purposes may not be the best for subsequent generalization and maintenance of trained behaviors.

The initial training of a target behavior is best accomplished with continuous reinforcement. In the early stages of training, most clients need a high density of reinforcement. Intermittent reinforcement schedules may be very inefficient at this stage. Generalization and maintenance of trained behaviors, on the other hand, are better promoted by an intermittent schedule. Therefore, after the behavior has been established to a certain extent by the use of continuous reinforcement, the clinician should switch to an intermittent schedule. When the target respones increase 30 to 50 percent over the baseline, continuous reinforcement may be discontinued. An FR2 may be appropriate to begin with. In gradual steps, the ratio may be increased.

SUMMARY

Within the treatment paradigm described in this book, the treatment variables available to speech-language clinicians are known as contingencies. A contingency describes a relation between certain stimulus conditions, a specified response, and the consequences that the clinician arranges for that response. One of the main clinical tasks is to create nonexisting communicative behaviors and increase the frequency of existing behaviors. A contingency helps the clinician accomplish this task.

One part of the treatment contingency deals with the behavior of the client, whereas two other parts deal with clinician behaviors. What the clinician does is treatment, and what the client does is the target. The clinician typically arranges stimulus conditions, which may include modeling, showing certain pictures, and so on. When the client begins to respond, the clinician arranges different consequences for correct and incorrect responses.

Consequences that help the client learn, increase, and maintain behaviors are known as reinforcers. There are two kinds of reinforcers: positive and negative.

Positive reinforcers are events that, when made contingent upon a response, increase the future rate of that response. Reinforcers are not defined in terms of subjective feelings and perceptions.

Five types of positive reinforcers were described: primary, social, conditioned generalized, informative feedback, and high probability behaviors. Each type of reinforcer has its strengths and weaknesses.

Primary reinforcers can be very effective, but they may not promote generalization of speech-language behaviors which are typically reinforced by social reinforcers. However, primary reinforcers may be necessary for clients who have limited verbal behaviors.

Social reinforcers are appropriate for reinforcing communicative behaviors. They minimize discrimination between treatment and natural environments.

Conditioned generalized reinforcers (tokens) are very desirable because they are not affected by satiation, but a variety of backup reinforcers is needed.

Informative feedback can be useful, but by itself it is a relatively weak reinforcer.

High probability behaviors can reinforce low probability behaviors. In using them as reinforcers, the clinician must control opportunities for exhibiting high probability behaviors.

Negative reinforcers are aversive events that, when terminated response contingently, can increase the rate of that response.

Escape and avoidance conditioning involves negative reinforcement. The clinical application of negative reinforcement has been limited.

A reinforcement schedule specifies a certain relation between responses, their number, or temporal characteristics on the one hand, and the reinforcer on the other.

In a continuous reinforcement schedule, reinforcers are presented for every response. This generates a high response rate that does not resist extinction well.

In a fixed ratio schedule, a predetermined number of responses is required for reinforcement. The schedule generates a high response rate with a postreinforcement pause.

In a variable ratio schedule, the number of responses required for reinforcement is varied around an average. A high and consistent response rate with no marked postreinforcement pause is the result.

A fixed interval schedule requires the passage of a fixed duration before a response can be reinforced. A relatively low response rate with distinct postreinforcement pauses is the result.

In a variable interval schedule, the time durations between reinforcers are allowed to vary around an average. The schedule generates a consistently high response rate with no pause after reinforcement.

The differential reinforcement of other behaviors is a schedule in which the behavior that will not be reinforced is specified. Many unspecified behaviors may be reinforced.

A continuous schedule must be used in the initial stages of clinical treatment, as this permits a faster acquisition of new responses. In subsequent stages of treatment, one of the several intermittent schedules is more appropriate. This can be expected to promote better generalization and maintenance of target behaviors.

STUDY GUIDE

Answer the following questions in technical language. Check your answers with the text. Rewrite your answers when necessary.

1. What are the two basic tasks of a speech-language pathologist?
2. What three factors are determined by consequences of responses?
3. Define reinforcement.
4. Define positive reinforcement.
5. What are some of the misunderstandings concerning positive reinforcers?
6. What is the single most critical criterion of defining positive reinforcers?
7. Name the five types of positive reinforcers.
8. Distinguish between primary and conditioned reinforcers.
9. Who might respond better to food as a reinforcer? Why?

10. What are the six limitations of food as a reinforcer?
11. Why are social reinforcers more appropriate in the treatment of communicative disorders?
12. What are the strengths and weaknesses of social reinforcers?
13. Define conditioned generalized reinforcers.
14. What is an everyday example of conditioned generalized reinforcers?
15. What are the different kinds of conditioned generalized reinforcers used in clinical situations?
16. What are the strengths and weaknesses of conditioned generalized reinforcers?
17. Define informative feedback and distinguish it from verbal reinforcers.
18. What is the most researched form of informative feedback?
19. What are EMGs, GSRs, and EEGs?
20. Describe the strengths and weaknesses of informative feedback.
21. Define high probability behaviors. What is another name for the same phenomenon?
22. Give some clinical examples of high probability behaviors.
23. What are the strengths and weaknesses of high probability behaviors?
24. What is the significance of "multiple contingencies"?
26. Define negative reinforcers. Give your own examples.
27. Distinguish between escape and avoidance. How are escape and avoidance behaviors reinforced?
28. What are schedules of reinforcement?
29. Define fixed and variable ratio schedules. Compare and contrast the two schedules in terms of their effects on response rates.
30. What is a postreinforcement pause? Under what schedules do you find it?
31. Define fixed and variable ratio schedules. Compare and contrast the two schedules in terms of their effects on response rates.
32. Write down everyday examples of reinforcement schedules.
33. What is a DRO? Define it with examples.
34. Write down clinical examples of the way each schedule can be used.
35. Why should you use intermittent schedules during the latter stages of training?

REFERENCES

Ayllon, T., and Azrin, N. H. (1968). *The token economy*. New York: Appleton-Century-Crofts.

Bailey, J. S., Timbers, G. D., Phillips, E. L., and Wolf, M. M. (1971). Modification of articulation errors of predelinquents by their peers. *Journal of Applied Behavior Analysis, 4,* 266–281.

Barrera, R. D., and Sulzer-Azaroff B. (1983). An alternating treatment comparison of oral and total communication training programs with echolalic autistic children. *Journal of Applied Behavior Analysis, 16,* 379–394.

Bennett, C. W. (1974). Articulation training in two hearing impaired girls. *Journal of Applied Behavior Analysis, 7,* 439–445.

Carr, E. G., and Kologinsky, E. (1983). Acquisition of sign language by autistic children. II: Spontaneity and generalization effects. *Journal of Applied Behavior Analysis, 16,* 297–314.

Campbell, C. and Stremel-Campbell, K. (1982). Programming "loose training" as a strategy to facilitate language generalization. *Journal of Applied Behavior Analysis, 15,* 295–301.

Elbert, M. and McReynolds, L. V. (1975). Transfer of /r/ across contexts. *Journal of Speech and Hearing Disorders, 40,* 380–387.

Ferster, C. B., and Skinner, B. F. (1957). *Schedules of reinforcement.* New York: Appleton-Century-Crofts.

Fitch, J. L. (1973). Voice and articulation. In B. B. Lahey (Ed.), *The modification of language behavior* (pp. 130–177). Springfield, IL: Charles C Thomas.

Flanagan, B., Goldiamond, I., and Azrin, N. H. (1958). Operant stuttering: The control of stuttering behavior through response-contingent consequences. *Journal of Applied Behavior Analysis, 1,* 173–177.

Guess, D., Sailor, W., Rutherford, G., and Baer, D. M. (1968). An experimental analysis of linguistic development: The productive use of the plural morpheme. *Journal of Applied Behavior Analysis, 1,* 225–235.

Hegde, M. N. (1979). Stuttering as operant behavior. *Journal of Speech and Hearing Research, 22,* 657–671.

Hegde, M. N., and Brutten, G. J, (1978). Reinforcing fluency in stutterers: An experimental study. *Journal of Fluency Disorders, 2,* 21–28.

Hegde, M. N. and Gierut, J. (1979). The operant training and generalization of pronouns and a verb form in a language delayed child. *Journal of Communication Disorders, 12,* 23–34.

Hegde, M. N. and McConn, J. (1981). Language training: Some data on response classes and generalization to an occupational setting. *Journal of Speech and Hearing Disorders, 46,* 353–358.

Hegde, M. N., Noll, M. J., and Pecora, R. (1979). A study of some factors affecting generalization of language training. *Journal of Speech and Hearing Disorders, 44,* 301–320.

Hurlbut, B. I., Iwata, B. A., & Green, J. D., (1982). Nonvocal language acquisition in adolescents with severe physical disabilities: Blissymbol versus iconic stimulus formats. *Journal of Applied Behavior Analysis, 15,* 241–258.

Ingham, R. J. (1984). *Stuttering and behavior therapy: Current status and experimental foundations.* San Diego, CA: College-Hill Press.

Ingham, R. J., Montgomery, J., and Ulliana, L. (1983). The effect of manipulating phonation duration on stuttering. *Journal of Speech and Hearing Research, 26,* 579–584.

Jackson, D. A. and Wallace, R. F. (1974). The modification and generalization of voice loudness in a fifteen-year old–retarded girl. *Journal of Applied Behavior Analysis, 7,* 461–471.

Johnston, J. M. and Johnston, G. T. (1972). Modification of consonant speech-sound articulation in young children. *Journal of Applied Behavior Analysis, 5*, 233–246.

Kazdin, A. E. (1984). *Behavior modification in applied settings* (3rd ed.). Homewood, IL: The Dorsey Press.

Mowrer, D. (1977). *Methods of modifying speech behaviors.* Columbus, OH: Charles E. Merrill.

Roll, D. (1973). Modification of nasal resonance in cleft-palate children by informative feedback. *Journal of Applied Behavior Analysis, 6*, 397–403.

Skinner, B. F. (1957). *Verbal behavior.* New York: Appleton-Century-Crofts.

Stevens-Long, J., and Rasmussen, M. (1974). The acquisition of simple and compound sentence structure in an autistic child. *Journal of Applied Behavior Analysis, 7*, 473–479.

Van Houten, R., and Nau, P. A. (1980). A comparison of the effects of fixed and variable ratio schedules of reinforcement on the behavior of deaf children. *Journal of Applied Behavior Analysis, 13*, 13–21.

Williams, G. C. and McReynolds, L. V. (1975). The relationship between discrimination and articulation training in children with misarticulation. *Journal of Speech and Hearing Research, 18*, 401–412.

Winokur, S. (1976). *A primer of verbal behavior: An operant view.* Englewood Cliffs, NJ.: Prentice-Hall.

Chapter 5

Treatment Programs I: The Basic Sequence

So far, an empirical and individual specific treatment program based on the concept of contingency has been discussed. In addition, procedures of documenting treatment effectiveness, selection and definition of target behaviors, and reinforcement schedules were described.

In Chapter 5, the following points will be described:

- A basic sequence of treatment that can be applied across various disorders of communication
- Establishing baselines of target behaviors before starting treatment
- Discrete trial-based training procedure
- Various criteria that suggest movement from one stage of training to the next
- An initial training and probe sequence

This chapter concerns how and in what sequence communicative disorders can be treated. At this point, it is assumed that the clinician has (1) interviewed the client and taken a history, (2) made an assessment of the client's communicative behaviors, (3) selected target behaviors to be trained, and (4) selected potential reinforcers to be used during the treatment sessions. The next step is to design and execute a treatment program.

Traditionally, treatment sessions are held immediately after an assessment is made. This follows the medical model in which diagnosis precedes treatment. In the current model, an assessment suggests only that there is a problem and that the client needs treatment. It can indicate potential target behaviors but cannot actually determine them. Since assessment involves a variety of activities, including interview and history taking, there is usually not enough time to measure client behaviors adequately. Absence of such pretreatment measures makes it difficult to establish treatment effectiveness, client improvement over time, and clinician accountability.

One way of overcoming the shortcomings of traditional assessment procedures is to establish baselines of target behaviors before treatment is started. The extra time spent on baselines can be worthwhile from the standpoint of reliability, clinician accountability, and the eventual evaluation of client improvement or treatment effectiveness.

An analysis of the client's assessment data suggests the possibility that multiple speech and language behaviors may be missing. All of those behaviors may be appropriate treatment targets. From a practical standpoint, the clinician can train only a few behaviors at a time. Because the baselines take a considerable amount of time, it is more efficient to baseline only those behaviors that will be trained immediately. Besides, valid baselines are those that are established just prior to treatment. Long time lapses between baselines and treatment may make it possible for extraneous variables to influence the target behaviors. Should this happen, the treatment effects cannot be evaluated, since dated baselines should not be used to determine treatment effects or client improvement over time.

BASELINES OF TARGET BEHAVIORS

Baselines can be defined as measured rates of behaviors in the absence of treatment. They can also be defined as the operant level of responses. In essence, baselines indicate the "natural," the typical, or the habitual rate of responses (Barlow, Hayes, and Nelson, 1984; Kazdin, 1984; Whaley and Malott, 1971). They help answer such questions as what percentage of a child's production of /s/ is correct, what percentage of words spoken by a client is stuttered, what percentage of the time a client speaks, whether he or she is able to sustain a certain voice quality, or how many manual signs a deaf individual can produce. In clinical terms, baselines are quantitative measures of correct and incorrect productions of communicative behaviors before treatment is initiated. In many cases, baselines may also be measures of a child's nonspeech behaviors, such as attending responses, in-seat behaviors, crying and whining, eye contact, or whatever. Any behavior the clinician plans to manipulate during treatment sessions needs to be baserated.

There are two basic reasons for establishing baselines before treatment. First, baselines give a reliable, valid measure of client behaviors prior to treatment. Unlike standardized tests, baselines involve adequate behavioral sampling. A given target behavior is evoked a number of times so that the client has had multiple opportunities to produce that behavior. Second, baselines make it possible to evaluate client improvement or treatment effectiveness. The response rates measured throughout the treatment sessions can be compared against the baselines to show that systematic changes in the client behaviors were associated with treatment.

Baseline Characteristics

Acceptable baselines should have at least two characteristics. First, baselines should be reliable. A reliable baseline is stable across time. Typically, the behaviors are measured repeatedly until some criterion of stability is reached. For example, one can say that the rate of stuttering measured in a client should not vary by more than 1 percent across two sessions. Similar criteria can be used in establishing baselines of articulatory, vocal, and language behaviors.

An exception to this criterion of stability is that a baseline showing a consistent worsening of the target behavior may be acceptable. This is known as a deteriorating baseline. It is acceptable because when a positive treatment effect is documented, it will have been unusually powerful in order to reverse a deteriorating trend in the target behavior.

Second, baselines should sample the target behaviors adequately. If they have to replace standardized test results, they must sample behaviors to a much greater extent than the tests do. For example, a standardized test of articulation may give the client two opportunities to produce the /s/ in the initial position of words. A baseline of the same behavior, however, may involve 20 words. Each word may also be presented on two trials. Thus, the actual number of opportunities to produce the /s/ may be 40, as against two or three on a standardized test. Similarly, the production of grammatic morphemes may be evoked in the context of 20 words or sentences, each presented on multiple trials.

It is often desirable to have a baseline measure of target behaviors exhibited in the client's everyday situations. Unfortunately, this is often not practical in routine clinical work. Whenever it is possible, extraclinical measures of target behaviors must be obtained. If the clinician is not able to measure target behaviors in the client's home or classroom, parents or teachers may be requested to tape record speech-language samples and submit them for analysis. In many cases, non-clinicians must be given some training in evoking and recording speech. Later, these measures can be used in assessing generalization.

Baseline Procedures

In establishing baselines of communicative behaviors, the following steps may be used. The steps are general enough to be applied across disorders. Necessary modifications can be made in case of specific disorders. Examples of several disorders are also given in order to illustrate the applicability of the steps across disorders.

Step 1: Specify the Target Behaviors. The first step is to have a clear idea of the behaviors to be baserated. If the client needs articulation training, the specific sounds or phonologic systems are specified. Another client may need language services, and the selected behaviors may be morphologic in nature. The number of dysfluencies exhibited by a stutterer may have to be reduced to 1 percent or less. A child with a repaired cleft may be initially trained in the nonnasal production of ten words that do not have any nasal sounds. All of these target behaviors are then operationally defined according to the criteria specified in Chapter 3. The clinician is then ready for the next step.

Step 2: Prepare the Stimulus Items. The second step in establishing baselines is to prepare stimulus items needed to evoke target responses. A variety of stimulus items can be prepared. Probably the most frequently used stimulus items are pictures. Typically, a specific picture is used in evoking a particular response. Real objects, whenever appropriate and convenient to use, should be selected as stimuli. Prior to more advanced stages of training, target behaviors may be baserated in conversational speech. In this case, the need for physical stimuli may be minimal.

The clients who need pictures or objects for stimuli are often children. The selected stimuli should be unambiguous and attractive. The pictures and objects should be appropriate for the particular child or client. Whenever possible, they should be selected from the client's natural environment. In many cases, pictures used in the initial stages of training may be simple in that they may depict single objects. Eventually, more complex pictures that evoke connected speech in the form of elaborate descriptions or stories may be needed.

Modeling the target responses can also be considered a form of stimulus. Frequently, clients in need of speech-language services, especially some young children, may not be able to give correct responses without the benefit of modeling. When the clinician models the correct response, the child may be able to imitate it. For this reason, modeling is used very frequently, especially in the early stages of training. The exact manner in which the target behavior is to be modeled must be predetermined.

When modeling is not to be used, the responses need to be evoked with the help of questions. Therefore, questions designed to evoke the specific target behaviors can also be considered stimuli, and must be prepared beforehand. Many target behaviors can be evoked with questions such as "what is this?" or "what do you see?" or "what is the boy doing?" or "where is the book?" But several other responses may require a more careful framing of questions so that the target behavior has the best chance of being evoked. Some target behaviors may need a combination of statements and questions. For example, in evoking a past tense inflection, one may have to say "Today, the man is walking. Yesterday, he did the same thing. What did he do yesterday? Yesterday he...." (Schumaker and Sherman, 1970). Still other behaviors may need a format in which no questions are asked, but a "sentence completion task" is required. For example, in evoking the regular plural morpheme /s/, the clinician may show a single object such as a book, and say "here is a book," and then point to two books, and say "here are two...." The client may be able to complete the sentence by saying "books" (Shipley and Banis, 1981).

In establishing baselines of target behaviors in conversational speech, open-ended requests or questions like "tell me about the picture" or "what is happening here?" or "what did you do this morning?" may be used. With adult clients, topic cards are often useful in maintaining conversational speech. On each index card, a specific topic of current interest or known to be of interest to the particular client can be written down. Several such cards can be prepared so that continuous speech can be evoked for extended periods of time.

About 20 stimulus items should be selected for each target behavior. If the /s/ is going to be trained in the initial position of words, 20 such words and corresponding pictures must be selected. Similar sets of words and pictures are needed for initial and medial positions. About the same number of stimulus items may be used in baserating morphologic features such as the present progressive *ing* or the preposition *on*. In this case, 20 words, phrases, or short sentences that include the target morpheme are used. If the clinician wishes to establish a baseline of "nasality," 20 words without nasal sounds may be used. Other vocal qualities may also be measured in similar ways.

In the initial stages of treatment, most target behaviors are taught at the simplest level of words and phrases. However, as mentioned before, the final target is the production of those behaviors in conversational speech used in everyday situations. For this reason, baselines of speech, language, voice, and fluency behaviors must be established at this level.

Step 3: Prepare a Recording Sheet. Since baselines are objectively measured rates of responses, each target response must be recorded on a recording sheet. This is in fact the most important step the clinician takes in establishing his or her accountability. Objectively recorded baselines can be compared later with response rates with and without treatment. They can also be used by independent observers to verify client improvement or treatment effectiveness. Therefore, it is necessary to design a recording sheet on which all responses are entered and scored.

Each clinician can design his or her own recording sheet and use it routinely. The format of the sheet should be flexible to accommodate differences in the way certain target behaviors are measured. Essentially, a recording sheet contains some basic information about the client and the clinician, a listing of the target behaviors, and spaces in which each of the client's attempts (trials) of every required response is in some way recorded. The sheet will also show whether each attempt was correct or incorrect, or whether the response was absent when one was required. An example of a recording sheet that can be modified by individual clinicians is given in Table 5–1.

The recording sheet illustrated in Table 5–1 shows how the production of the plural morpheme /s/ was baserated in the context of 20 words. Each of the 20 target responses was presented on two discrete trials, which will shortly be described. The clinician then recorded correct, incorrect, and no responses. Finally, the percent correct response rate was calculated. This particular client was able to produce the plural morpheme in single words with 20 percent accuracy when evoked, and with 45 percent accuracy when modeled. As can be seen, such statements are stronger than those based on standardized tests of language performance, which often do not yield percent correct response rates.

The recording sheet could just as easily illustrate a baseline of an articulatory behavior. A client's production of /z/, for example, can be baserated in the context of single words by use of the same two-trial procedure. Each production is judged as correct or incorrect and marked accordingly. The clinician can then calculate the percent correct response rate for the production of /z/. Similarly, vocal characteristics such as nasality or hoarseness observed while the client produces selected utterances can be recorded on the sheet as long as

Table 5–1.   Illustration of a Two-Trial Baseline Recording Sheet

Client:	Clinician:
Age:	Date:
Disorders: language	Session No.
Target behavior: plural /s/	Reinforcement: noncontingent

	Trials	
Target Behaviors	**Evoked**	**Modeled**
1. Cups	−	+
2. Boots	−	−
3. Hats	−	+
4. Plates	−	−
5. Bats	+	+
6. Ducks	−	−
7. Ships	−	+
8. Cats	+	+
9. Boats	−	−
10. Rabbits	−	−
11. Coats	−	+
12. Nuts	0	−
13. Goats	−	−
14. Plants	−	−
15. Blocks	+	+
16. Lamps	0	0
17. Rats	−	−
18. Ants	−	+
19. Trucks	+	+
20. Pots	−	−

Note: (+) = correct   (−) = incorrect   (0) = no response

Correct production of the plural morpheme:
Evoked: 20 percent   Modeled: 45 percent

Specified target behaviors can be any measurable behavior at any topography (words, phrases, sentences).

each attempt on the part of the client is treated as a discrete trial. Under the heading "target behaviors," words, phrases, or sentences can be written. This makes it possible to baserate a majority of communicative behaviors selected for training.

In recording the baselines of target behaviors in conversational speech, the clinician may not use the format illustrated in Table 5–1, which is most suitable for a discrete-trial procedure. Conversational speech is typically recorded (audio or video) for later analysis.

Step 4: Administer the Baseline Trials. It was mentioned earlier that stimulus items are administered on discrete trials. Our recording sheet shows that each target response was administered on one evoked and one modeled trial. The difference between these two kinds of trials is the presence or the absence of modeling by the clinician. On an evoked trial the clinician simply asks a question and expects the client to respond. The outcome in terms of correct, incorrect, or no response is recorded. On an evoked trial, the clinician asks a question but does not model the correct response. For example, in baserating the regular plural /s/, the clinician might show the client selected pictures of plural objects. Immediately, the clinician might ask questions such as "what do you see?" or "what are these?" The client might say "cup" (or "cups"), "book" (or "books"), and so on. Such trials are called evoked because of the absence of modeling by the clinician.

A modeled trial, on the other hand, is designed to find out if a response not typically produced by the client is imitated. Soon after asking the question "what are these?" the clinician will add "say, two cups." The clinician should probably add the client's name to the modeled response ("John, say, two cups"). If the client were to say "two cups," it is then scored as a correctly imitated response. It is useful to know if the client can imitate the target behaviors. If there is no imitation, then the client must be taught to imitate. If the client can imitate, this step can be skipped. In addition, when multiple responses are baserated, those that are imitated correctly (but not produced on evoked trials) can be trained first.

A third sequence of evoked trial (not illustrated in Table 5–1) may occasionally be used to informally evaluate the effects of the previous modeled trial. A client who did not produce a particular response on the first evoked trial but did produce it on the modeled trial may sometimes be successful on a subsequent evoked trial. This would give additional information on the relative ease with which baselined responses can be trained. An additional set of evoked trials would extend the time spent on baselines, and therefore may not be used all the time.

What is a trial? A trial is a structured opportunity to produce a given target response with or without modeling. Trials are discrete when they are temporally separated from one another. A trial consists of a sequence of interdependent events. These events are a part of the behavioral contingency discussed earlier.

The steps involved in administering a discrete evoked trial are as follows:

1. Place the stimulus picture in front of the client, or demonstrate the action or event with the help of objects.
2. Ask the relevant question, which has been predetermined.
3. Wait a few seconds for the client to respond.
4. Record the response on the recording sheet.
5. Pull the picture toward you, or remove it from the subject's view.
6. Wait 2 or 3 seconds to mark the end of the trial.

The clinician goes back to step one to initiate the next trial.

A modeled trial is administered as follows:

1. Place the stimulus picture in front of the client, or demonstrate the action or event with the help of objects.
2. Ask the predetermined question.
3. Immediately, model the correct response ("Johnny, say...").
4. Wait a few seconds for the client to respond.
5. Record the response on the recording sheet.
6. Pull the picture toward you, or remove it from the subject's view.
7. Wait 2 or 3 seconds to mark the end of the trial.

The next trial is soon initiated by placing the picture in front of the client. It may be noted that the evoked and the modeled trials are similar except for the clinician's modeling on the latter. It is helpful to have the picture stimuli neatly stacked so that one picture at a time is pulled out and presented to the client. Scattered stimulus materials tend to evoke competing responses from young children. The children may respond to multiple stimuli simultaneously, making it difficult to measure individual responses.

In order to measure responses on discrete trials, it is necessary to move or remove the picture at the end of the trial. That helps sepa-rate each attempt on the part of the client and also prevents the client from responding before the clinician asks the relevant question or models. The procedure can also help record individual responses, because it can regulate the clinician's behavior as well.

Reinforcement in a Baseline Sequence

By definition, baselines are response rates in the absence of the treatment variable. As such, the reinforcement contingency, con-sidered the treatment variable in the paradigm presented in Chapter 1, cannot be imposed on correct behaviors. Nor can a punishing con-tingency be imposed on incorrect responses. In the absence of contin-gent consequences, the clinician should simply evoke and record the responses. However, most baselines require many responses from a client. Sometimes, three or four target behaviors are baserated. This can create a motivational problem for some clients, especially for the young. They may not continue to respond in the absence of reinforcement.

One way of handling the motivational problem during baseline sessions is to reinforce the client in a noncontingent manner. Periodically, the client may be reinforced for "doing a fine job," "good sitting," "looking at the picture," or "saying the words." These reinforcers are not contingent upon correct target responses being measured. Therefore, every reinforcer is presented during a brief pause so that there is no contingency between responses and the consequence. For the young child, these reinforcing occasions may also provide some needed breaks from structured trials. Such noncontingent reinforcers may also be given when the target behaviors are baserated in conversational speech or oral reading.

ANALYSIS OF BASELINE DATA

Baseline data are analyzed to arrive at a percent correct response rate. The recording sheet illustrated earlier showed the percent correct response rates for the production of the plural morpheme. The measure can be calculated for the production of various speech sounds. The percentage of syllables stuttered or percentage of words stuttered can be calculated at the level of words, phrases, or sentences. Vocal qualities can also be analyzed in terms of either the time duration for which a given quality was sustained, or the number of words, phrases, or sentences produced with the appropriate vocal target. In turn, a percent correct score can be calculated for these measures.

The percent correct response rate can also be calculated when target behaviors are measured in the conversational speech mode. Frequencies of correct and incorrect productions of phonemes can be counted in conversational speech. The number of times a grammatic feature is used correctly can be counted, along with the number of times it is required but not used. Similarly, frequencies of stuttering behaviors, along with the number of words spoken, can be observed. The number of words (or syllables) on which pitch breaks occurred can be recorded, along with those on which desirable pitch was sustained. Such measures allow calculations of percent correct response rates.

The frequency with which a given communicative behavior is exhibited is probably the most objective of the measures available to clinicians. Absolute number of responses and percent correct response rates are preferable to subjective statements because they are easily verified by other clinicians.

THE BASIC TREATMENT PROGRAM

From a conceptual standpoint, treatment involves effecting changes in the client's communicative behaviors. Often, certain non-verbal behaviors such as uncooperative responses need to be changed as well. By systematic arrangement of appropriate contingencies, the clinician can accomplish these tasks.

The treatment procedure described in this chapter is based on the treatment paradigm described in Chapter 1. Experimental-clinical research has been done for more than two decades on the efficacy of the behaviorial treatment procedures in communicative disorders. In the treatment of many behavior disorders unrelated to speech and language, the evidence has a much longer history. More importantly, these clinical procedures are based upon principles enunciated by replicated laboratory research.

The procedures have been used extensively in the habilitation or rehabilitation of a variety of clinical populations, including the mentally retarded, emotionally disturbed, brain injured, autistic, behaviorally disordered, and hearing impaired. The procedures have also been used successfully in regular and special educational classrooms. The interested reader should consult some of the annual series of publications, such as the one edited by Hersen, Eisler, and Miller entitled *Progress in Behavior Modification*.

Experimental Foundations of the Treatment Program

A comprehensive analysis of verbal behavior in terms of experimentally established controlling contingencies was published by Skinner in 1957. Following this, some of the earliest applications of behavioral methodology in the field of speech were done in the area of infant vocalization (Rheingold, Gewirtz, and Ross, 1959; Todd and Palmer, 1968; Weisberg, 1961). These studies showed (and subsequent studies confirmed) that infant vocalizations can be increased or decreased by appropriate behavioral contingencies (Schumaker and Sherman, 1978).

One of the earliest disorders of communication to be researched with the behavioral methodology was stuttering. In 1958, Flanagan,

Goldiamond, and Azrin demonstrated that stuttering could be brought under the influence of reinforcing as well as punishing contingencies. This study stimulated a series of investigations on stuttering within the conditioning and learning framework. Many studies, both experimental and treatment oriented, have been published and still continue to be published (Brutten, 1975; Costello, 1980; Gray and England, 1969; Hegde, 1978, 1979, 1985; Hegde and Brutten, 1977; Ingham, 1984; Martin, 1968; Martin and Siegel, 1966; Mowrer, 1979; Ryan, 1974; Shames and Florence, 1980; Shames and Sherrick, 1963).

Systematic behavioral treatment of language disorders was initiated during the 1960s and early 1970s, when Chomskyan transformational grammar was very popular. During this time the nativists (Chomsky, 1957, 1965; Lenneberg, 1967; McNeil, 1970) had raised serious questions about the possibility of empirical manipulations of language. The suggestion was that languages are innately determined and that therefore behavioral or other environmental manipulations may not have significant effects on them. A majority of early experimental studies in the area of language disorders demonstrated that language was susceptible to the influence of the behavioral contingency, as stated by Skinner (1957). Most of these early studies were done on language disorders associated with mentally retarded and autistic children. Many of the pioneering studies were done by Baer, Guess, Sailor, Rutherford, and their colleagues in the treatment of mentally retarded subjects and by Lovaas and his colleagues in the treatment of autistic children (Guess, 1969; Guess and Baer, 1973a; Guess, Sailor, Rutherford, and Baer, 1968; Lovaas, 1966; Sailor, Guess, Rutherford, and Baer, 1968).

Subsequently, operant training of language disordered children and adults became well established. In fact, the treatment of language disorders based upon the principles of instructions, modeling, differential reinforcement, shaping, fading, and generalization or maintenance is probably the most tested of language training procedures available today. This is because numerous studies have produced controlled evidence in support of behavioral treatment techniques (Campbell and Stremel-Campbell, 1982; Connell and McReynolds, 1981; Costello, 1983; Garcia and DeHaven, 1974; Guess and Baer, 1973b; Guess, Sailor, and Baer, 1978; Gray and Ryan, 1971, 1973; Harris, 1975; Hegde, 1980; Hegde and Gierut, 1979; Hegde and McConn, 1981; Hegde, Noll, and Pecora, 1979; Koegel and Rincover, 1977; McDonald and Blott, 1974; McReynolds, 1974; Risley and Wolf, 1967; Schumaker and Sherman, 1970; Welch, 1981, among others).

Behavioral technology has also been demonstrated to be effective in the treatment of articulation disorders. Essentially the same techniques of contingency management have been able to effect changes in articulatory behaviors of children and adults (Bailey, Timbers, Phillips, and Wolf, 1971; Baker and Ryan, 1971; Bennett, 1974; Costello, 1977; Costello and Onstine, 1976; Elbert and McReynolds, 1975; Fitch, 1973; Holland and Mathews, 1963; Johnston and Johnston, 1972; McReynolds and Elbert, 1981; Mowrer, 1977; Mowrer, Baker, and Schutz, 1968; Williams and McReynolds, 1975; among others).

There are relatively few studies on the behavioral treatment of voice disorders. Nevertheless, they have demonstrated that voice disorders as well as normal vocal behaviors can be modified by the same procedures as those used in the behavioral treatment of language, articulation, and fluency disorders (Blake and Moss, 1967; Fitch, 1973; Fleece, Gross, O'Brien, Kistner, Rothblum, and Drabman, 1981; Jackson and Wallace, 1974; Lane, 1964; Moore and Holbrook, 1971; Patterson, Teigen, Liberman, and Austin, 1975; Roll, 1973; Schwartz and Hawkins, 1970, among others).

Teaching nonverbal communication (sign language) to profoundly retarded, autistic, and hearing impaired individuals has also been researched within the behavioral paradigm. A number of excellent studies are now available. In addition to teaching sign language, the investigators have addressed many aspects of habilitation and rehabilitation of such populations (Barrera and Sulzer-Azaroff, 1983; Carr, 1979, 1982; Carr, Binkoff, Kologinsky, and Eddy, 1978; Carr and Kologinsky, 1983; Duker and Morsink, 1984; Faw, Reid, Schepis, Fitzgerald, and Welty, 1981; Hurlbut, Iwata, and Green, 1982; Remington and Clark, 1983; among others).

The treatment procedure to be described here is based upon extensive laboratory and clinical research of the kind just cited.

THE BASIC TREATMENT PROCEDURE

In this section, an essential sequence of treatment is outlined. The sequence can be altered at different stages of treatment, and to suit individual clients and disorders. The sequence includes various objective criteria by which movement throughout the program and eventual progress of the client can be determined. In a Chapter 9, some advanced features of the training program will be described.

The discrete trial procedure, used in establishing baselines, is also used in training target behaviors. Most of the studies cited earlier illustrate many aspects of the procedure to be described. A study by Hegde, Noll, and Pecora (1979) provides a specific illustration of the procedure as applied in language training.

The training sequence is initiated after the target behaviors are baserated. They are often trained one at a time, although in some cases, two or three behaviors can be trained in single sessions. In either case, training on a given response is started at the level of a word, a phrase, or a sentence. In the initial stage of training, most clients need modeling. Therefore, the training trial is very similar to the modeled baseline trials except that it includes the treatment variable.

The treatment variable is the specific consequence programmed for the target responses. Positive reinforcement contingencies are placed on the production of desirable target responses. Contingencies of extinction and punishment are placed on behaviors that need to be decreased. It is important to note that the extinction and punishment contingencies, described fully in a later chapter, are as important as the reinforcing contingencies.

A training trial is also a sequence of events that includes certain actions on the part of the client and the clinician. A typical discrete training trial in which modeling is included has the following steps:

1. Place the stimulus item in front of the client, or demonstrate the action or event with the help of objects.
2. Ask the predetermined question.
3. Immediately, model the correct response.
4. Wait a few seconds for the client to respond.
5. If the client's response is correct, reinforce it immediately by verbal praise and any other potential reinforcer.
6. If the client's response is incorrect, punish it immediately.
7. Record the response on the recording sheet.
8. Pull the stimulus item toward you, or remove it from the client's view.
9. Wait a few seconds to mark the end of the trial.

The next trial is then initiated by placing the picture again in front of the client.

In some forms of stuttering and voice treatment, presentation of pictures and objects may not be necessary. The treatment may be started with one word or two word responses modeled or evoked by the clinician. Questions that evoke single responses may be asked, and if necessary, the response may be modeled immediately. However, each attempt on the part of the client is treated as a discrete trial, and responses are measured accordingly.

When modeling is discontinued, training continues on evoked discrete trials. The sequence of events is the same as that just specified, except that the clinician does not model (step 3 would be omitted).

The client is given a chance to respond appropriately to the question asked by the clinician.

When the client begins to imitate the correct response more consistently, the clinician must discontinue modeling. When to do this is one of the early "choice points" the clinician is likely to face. The clinician needs an objective criterion by which this decision can be made. A criterion of five consecutively correct imitated responses can serve this purpose. In other words, when the client imitates correctly on five consecutive trials, modeling is discontinued and the evoked trials are initiated.

When evoked trials are introduced the first time, the correct response may or may not be produced by the client. Initially, a lack of modeling may lead to incorrect responses or no responses at all. Should this happen, the clinician needs to reintroduce modeling. Once again, the clinician must have an objective criterion to make this decision. According to a criterion used in some studies, modeling can be reintroduced when the correct responses are not observed on two or three consecutive evoked trials. Modeling can be continued until five consecutively correct imitated responses are noted again. As before, evoked trials are reintroduced at this point.

It can be expected that eventually the client will emit correct responses on evoked trials with increasing consistency. Soon, the clinician must judge whether the first training item (a word, phrase, or sentence) has been tentatively trained. The training must move on to the next item. An objectively specified training criterion will help the clinician in this regard. A training criterion specifies how many correct responses must be recorded consecutively before the response can be considered tentatively learned. A range of 10 to 20 consecutive correct responses (sometimes recorded across two consecutive sessions) has been required by most clinicians.

When the client reaches the adopted training criterion on the first item, the second item is picked up for training. Starting with the first trial, modeling is provided until the client emits four to five consecutively correct imitated responses. Evoked trials would then be introduced. If necessary, modeling is reintroduced at any time according to the above mentioned criterion. Training will continue until the client reaches the training criterion.

Management of Treatment Contingencies

The most important factor in administering treatment trials is to manage the reinforcing and punishing contingencies. The correct response, whether imitated or evoked, must be reinforced immediately.

There should be no hesitation in the delivery of reinforcement. Some clinicians hesitate because they have trouble judging whether the response was correct or not. Consequently, the intended reinforcing consequence may be delayed and ambiguous. A statement or type of consequence such as "maybe it was OK; I will let you have this," may not be effective. Sometimes, the clinician may first record the response and then reinforce it. This also causes delayed reinforcement. Such delays are undesirable, especially in the beginning stage of training. The clinician must be able to judge the accuracy of the response instantaneously and reinforce immediately.

Another potential problem is a weak (too soft, unsure) and monotonous delivery of verbal praise. Verbal reinforcers such as "good" and "I like that" may be uttered without any affect, smile, or appropriate facial expressions. Although there is no controlled evidence on this issue, such mechanical delivery of verbal praise may not be effective. Verbal praise must be strong, natural, and full of affect. It must be accompanied by appropriate facial expressions and other gestures.

The punishing consequencs must also be delivered promptly for incorrect responses. A hesitant and weak "no" may be as ineffective as a delayed and affectless "good." This means that the clinician must be quick in identifying and punishing wrong and uncooperative responses (see Chapter 8 for details).

The clinician should also remember all the time that the selected consequence may or may not act as reinforcers or punishers. The response rate must be measured continuously so that the effect of consequent events can be monitored. When the target responses do not change, the consequences must be changed.

Number of Individual Responses to be Trained

With the procedure just described, the clinician can train additional responses of the first target behavior. Soon, a decision must be made regarding the termination of training on the first target behavior and moving on to the next. The clinician must base this decision on some empirical data, not on subjective judgment. When a behavior is learned by the client is a question that can be answered on some empirical grounds. In a final sense, a target behavior is learned when it is produced by the client in his or her natural environment under normal conditions of stimuli and consequences. For continued responding, there should be no need for pictures, modeling, prompts, and other stimuli. Also, the response rate should be maintained with the types and amounts of reinforcers available in the natural environment. In short, a target response has met the final dismissal criterion when its maintenance in everyday situations has been documented. This dismissal criterion might specify a correct response rate of at least 90 percent in conversational speech in everyday situations. Therefore, as many responses as are needed to achieve this criterion must be trained.

The final dismissal criterion is not realized in the early part of training. In fact, it may not be realized until special maintenance procedures are implemented. This will need additional time and planning. Meanwhile, the clinician has the other selected target behaviors to train. Therefore, within the training sequence, only a limited generalization is assessed to determine the need for additional training on the target behavior being taught at any given time. When most of the target behaviors are trained to a certain level of proficiency, a program of response maintenance may be initiated. In essence, then, the clinician needs a tentative criterion by which the decision to go on to the next target behavior can be made. This is done with the realization that most probably additional training and maintenance strategies must be implemented later.

The decision to move on to the next target behavior is made on the basis of a tentative probe criterion. A probe is a procedure designed to assess the generalized production of a trained target behavior. The final probe criterion assesses the generalized production of the target behaviors in conversational speech produced in the client's natural environments. On the other hand, tentative probe criteria are many and are defined in the program. There may be different tentative probes implemented at different stages of treatment. In the very first stage, for example, the initial probe criterion may require that in order to move on to the next target behavior, the clinician must obtain a 90 percent correct production of the behavior being trained in the context of selected untrained words, phrases, or sentences. Obviously, this type of generalization is limited. Nevertheless, it may be sufficient to temporarily terminate the training on a given target behavior and initiate training on the next.

To summarize, when a target behavior meets an initial probe criterion of 90 percent correct, the clinician can start the training on the next target behavior. The 90 percent accuracy may be measured at the level of words, phrases, or sentences, depending upon the level of training.

Thus far, the training sequence described involved the training of individual stimulus items of the first target behavior. Perhaps the clinician has trained three or four responses under the first target behavior. At this time, the clinician should probably probe to see if the initial (tentative) probe criterion can be met. If so, the treatment can be initiated on the next target behavior. We should therefore describe the initial probe procedure.

The Initial Probe Procedure

The initial probe procedure is administered as soon as the client has met the training criterion on a certain number of stimulus items. Sometimes, the probe is administered after four responses of a given target behavior have been taught. In the case of plural /s/, for example, probing may be done after the client has met the training criterion on each of the following four responses: *cups, boots, hats,* and *plates.* It may be noted parenthetically that in the terminology used here, the class of plural /s/ production is a target behavior, and a specific plural word, phrase, or sentence is a particular response. At other times, probes may be administered after only two responses are trained. As a general rule, probes should be implemented after four to six items have been trained. There is some evidence that in language training, four to six stimulus items may be sufficient to obtain an initial, within-clinic generalization on structured probe trials (Guess and Baer, 1973b; Hegde, Noll, and Pecora, 1979). However, other behaviors such as fluency or voice or articulation may require additional training before generalization is assessed in the clinic. Clinicians should not hesitate to experiment with this suggested criterion of four to six training items before initiating a probe sequence.

Because probes are designed to assess the production of untrained responses, stimulus items that were not used in training must be presented on the probe trials. You may recall that in the beginning the clinician will have developed at least 20 stimulus items for each target behavior. If, for a particular target behavior, six of them have been used in the training process, the clinician can now use the remaining 16 untrained stimulus items to probe generalization.

Probes are also administered on discrete trials. However, responses given on the probe trials are not reinforced. Thus, the probe trials are similar to the baseline trials. Consequently, massed probe trials can create motivational problems for young clients. It may be difficult to have the child respond for prolonged periods of time in the absence of reinforcers; actually, the trained responses may be extinguished. Therefore, a probe in which the already trained items are also used is preferred. This type is called an interspersed or intermixed probe. Intermixed probes are typically used in the initial and intermediate stages of treatment.

In an intermixed probe sequence, correct responses given to the trained stimulus items are reinforced, while those given to the probe items are not. Incorrect responses on trained items are also handled the way they were during training. They may be punished or ignored. This procedure is implemented to discourage discriminated response rates on trained and untrained items. In effect, the intermixed probe prevents the client from experiencing an extinction schedule.

A probe in which only the untrained items are presented is called a pure probe. Pure probes may be appropriate when the client is about to be dismissed. By this time, the clinician will have implemented several procedures to build up resistance to extinction. The amount of reinforcement will have been reduced gradually by using progressively larger ratios. Certain kinds of reinforcers may have been completely withdrawn. Family members may have been trained to provide a certain level of reinforcement at home and other situations. Because of these and other procedures, the client's response rates will have been maintained in the absence of heavy, continuous reinforcement. Therefore, at the time of dismissal, the client can be expected to sustain the response rate on a pure probe.

In administering an intermixed probe, the clinician keeps the already trained stimulus items in one pile and the untrained stimulus items in another pile. Individual stimulus items from the two sets are alternated. On the initial trial, a trained stimulus item may be presented, just as on any training trial. The second trial, however, is different, because on this trial, an untrained stimulus item is presented. The predetermined question is asked, and a few seconds are allowed for the client to respond. The response is simply recorded, with no contingent consequences (reinforcers or punishers). In other words, the actual probe trial is identical to the baseline trial. Thus, trained and untrained items are presented on alternating trials in an intermixed probe sequence.

No modeling is provided on any of the probe trials. Trained and untrained stimulus items are presented on evoked trials only. As a result, most probes have a single set of trials.

In later stages of training, probes may not involve any discrete trials. When the target behaviors have been trained in conversational speech, probes should sample generalized response rates in this response mode. In Chapter 7, procedures designed to enhance and assess generalization and maintenance will be described.

Although the probe trial is identical to the baseline trial, it is not called that for two reasons. First, the purpose of the baseline trial is to establish the operant level of a response, whereas the purpose of a probe trial is to assess generalized production of the trained response. Second, the two sets of trials are administered at different times in the training program. Whereas the baselines are administered before the treatment is started, the probes are administered after the behavior has been trained to a certain extent. In essence, the baselines assess the rate of behavior in the absence of treatment, whereas the probes assess certain effects of treatment. For these reasons, it is necessary to keep the two terms separate.

Analysis of Probe Results

In the analysis of probe results, the trials involving trained stimuli are ignored, and only the responses evoked by untrained stimuli are included. The purpose of the analysis is to determine the percent correct generalized response rate. The same procedure that is used in calculating the correct response rate on the baseline trials can be used here. The number of probe stimulus items presented, and the number of correct responses given by the client, are counted, and the percent correct response rate is derived.

The next step to be taken by the clinician depends on the recorded probe response rate. You may recall that as a general rule, a probe is administered when four to six items are trained to the training criterion. The results of this probe will determine whether additional training is needed for the same target behavior, or the next target behavior can now be trained. The clinician needs an objective criterion by which to make this decision. In some clinical studies, a criterion of 90 percent correct response rate on probe trials has been used. This is one of the several probe criteria used in different stages of treatment.

If the initial probe response rate is at least 90 percent correct, then the next target behavior can be trained. However, some of the treatment time can also be spent on training the same target behavior at a higher level of response topography. For example, if the first target behavior trained at the level of single words has met the 90 percent correct probe response rate, then the training may be shifted to a two word phrase level. When the behavior meets the probe criterion at one of the higher levels of response topography (such as conversational speech in the clinic), then a program of maintenance can be initiated so that the target behavior can be produced in the client's natural environment. Such additional training or maintenance programs can be implemented while the second or the third target behavior is being trained at lower levels of response complexity.

If the probed response rate falls short of the 90 percent correct probe criterion, then additional training is needed for the same target behavior. While the first behavior is still being trained, the clinician can spend a portion of the treatment time on the next target behavior, however.

Additional Training for the Previously Trained Behavior

There are two ways in which additional training can be provided for a behavior that fails to meet the initial probe criterion. If the observed probe response rate is relatively low (70 percent or less), additional stimulus items can be selected for further training. On the other hand, if the recorded probe response rate is in excess of 70 percent, then a series of additional training trials on the already trained items may be sufficient to obtain a 90 percent correct response rate on the next probe.

If additional trials on the previously trained behavior do not improve the correct response rate on the next probe, it is probably best to pick up new stimulus items for further training. After training several new stimulus items, a probe can be conducted again.

In essence, training and probe procedures are alternated until the 90 percent correct probe response rate is achieved. There is no fixed number of stimulus items that when trained will assure generalization of target behaviors in all clients. In fact, the amount of training needed will vary greatly across individual clients. The probe criterion provides the clinician with an objective and flexible way of making decisions regarding the amount of training needed in given cases. The clinician should perhaps avoid the temptation of probing too soon, because probes consume time that may be better used in training. On the other hand, excessive training at a single level of response topography must be avoided. Such training, especially at single word level, may be inefficient because the training must move on to more complex levels, to the next target behavior, or both. Relatively frequent probes, when successful, can help make transitions in the treatment sequence at appropriate times.

Treatment of the Second and the Subsequent Target Behaviors

As has been suggested, the clinician need not wait until the first target behavior has reached the final dismissal criterion to initiate treatment on the second target behavior. Actually, in many cases, two or three target behaviors can be trained in the same treatment session. For example, more than one phoneme can be trained in the initial stage of articulation therapy. In language disorders, two or three response classes can be trained in the same treatment session. In the treatment of stuttering, oral reading and speech (at some level) may be simultaneously targeted for treatment. Similarly, a voice disorder can be treated at the level of oral reading and spontaneous utterances of limited response topography.

On the other hand, the clinician may wish to focus upon a single target behavior in the initial stages of treatment. With some clients, a single target may be desirable because it may result in a relatively rapid progress. This may have a beneficial effect upon the client's motivation. The initial target behavior may have had a higher baseline level, making it somewhat easier to teach than the other behaviors with low operant levels. Responses of a low operant level may be better taught at a later stage. However, when two or three target behaviors are of relatively high operant level, they can all be selected for initial treatment. The sessions then can have some stimulus and response variety.

The sequence of treatment depends upon the number of behaviors being taught initially. If only one target behavior is being trained, then a successful probe may suggest two possibilities that are not mutually exclusive. First, the treatment can be shifted to a higher level of response complexity involving the same target behavior. Second, the treatment can be started on the next target behavior while the first one continues to be trained at a more complex level of response topography. When multiple target behaviors are trained simultaneously, a successful probe on any behavior should lead to training at more complex levels of response topography.

When the initial, in-the-clinic, structured probe criterion is achieved for the selected behaviors, the clinician can implement training on additional target behaviors, initiate a maintenance program on already trained behaviors, or both.

AN EXAMPLE OF INITIAL TRAINING AND PROBE SEQUENCE

The training procedure, stages of treatment, probe sequence, and various criteria just described are illustrated here. The client is a six year old child named Tommy with a language disorder. After the

Table 5-2. Summary of Hypothetical Baseline Data on a Six Year Old Language Disordered Child

Client: Tommy Logos	Clinician: Linda Verbose
Age: 6 years	Date: September 10, 1985
Disorder: language	Session No. 2
Target behaviors: Plural /s/, aux. "is", prep., "on" and (reg) past tense /d/	Reinforcement: Noncontingent, verbal

Target Behaviors	Evoked	Modeled (Percent Correct Responses)
1. The plural /s/ (cups, boots, etc.)	31	37
2. The auxiliary "is" (boy is running, boy is jumping, etc.)	18	30
3. The preposition "on" (on table, on chair, etc.)	9	10
4. Regular past tense /d/ (she opened, she pulled, etc.)	0	4

Note: All error responses involved omission of the target feature.

Each of the target behaviors was baserated with 20 stimulus items

assessment, the clinician baserated the following four grammatic features: the plural /s/, the auxiliary *is*, the preposition *on*, and the regular past tense ending with /d/. Each behavior was baserated with 20 stimulus items on a set of evoked trials, and a set of modeled trials according to the procedure illustrated in Table 5-1. The percent correct response rate varied from 0 to 37. Table 5-2 summarizes the hypothetical baseline data for this client. Appendix A illustrates the treatment data recording procedure. It shows only the first six stimulus items of the initial target behavior.

The plural /s/ was trained first. Treatment was started at the level of single words. The first word trained was "cups." To begin with, the clinician modeled the correct response. A picture of two cups was placed in front of the child, and the clinician asked the question "what are these?" and immediately modeled the correct response by saying "Tommy, say cups." The recording sheet (Appendix A) shows that the response was scored incorrect. Perhaps the child said "cup" as he had done on the baseline trials. The clinician immediately said "no" and recorded the response as incorrect (−) on the recording sheet. The picture was pulled toward the clinician, and after a few seconds the next trial was initiated.

Often, an emphasis on the target response will help the client imitate it. Thus, the clinician emphasized the /s/ in the word "cups" in order to focus upon the target response. Tommy imitated the response on the second modeled trial, and the clinician immediately reinforced it verbally. A token was also given. An accumulation of 15 tokens would give Tommy two minutes of play with a toy of his choice. The clinician recorded the response and pulled the stimulus picture away from the child. After a few seconds, the third trial was initiated. The recording sheet shows that this type of discrete trial procedure continued until Tommy gave five consecutively correct imitated responses. In the beginning, the numbers of correct and incorrect responses were about equal, but soon more correct than incorrect responses were emitted. Tommy needed 18 trials before he could imitate the response on four successive trials.

The evoked trial was introduced on trial 19 by omitting modeling. According to the recording sheet, Tommy's responses on the first two evoked trials (numbered 19 and 20) were wrong. They were verbally punished by a "no." Modeling was reinstated on trial 21. The next five responses were correctly imitated (trials 21 to 25). Therefore, modeling was once again discontinued on the 26th trial. This time, Tommy's response on the evoked trial was correct. Occasionally, however, incorrect responses were given, but they became less frequent. Ten consecutively correct evoked responses (the training criterion) were eventually recorded. The recording sheet shows that Tommy needed a total of 47 trials to reach that training criterion.

The clinician then initiated training on the next response ("boots"). Once again, modeling was used in the beginning. This time Tommy readily imitated the response. The responses were correct on the first five modeled trials, and therefore, the sixth was an evoked trial. Tommy's response on this trial was wrong, but it was correct on the next trial. Once again, correct and incorrect responses were interspersed to begin with, but gradually an increase in the rate of the correct response was noted. Tommy reached the training criterion of ten consecutively correct responses in 28 trials.

Four more responses, "hats," "plates," "bats," and "ducks," were trained in the same manner. As the recording sheet shows, the number of incorrect responses showed a progressive decrease as the training continued. Tommy was able to give correct responses from the beginning on the last two training items, with only two incorrect responses each.

After Tommy achieved the training criterion on the sixth response, the clinician probed for generalization. The remaining 14 baselined stimulus items (not used in training) were presented on an intermixed probe sequence. Starting with a trained item, trained and untrained items were alternated on consecutive trials. The responses given to already trained stimulus items were all correct and were reinforced. Some of the responses given to the probe (untrained) items were correct and others were incorrect, but they were neither reinforced nor punished. The first probe showed a correct response rate of 64 percent. This generalized response rate did not meet the probe criterion and thus indicated a need for additional training. The probe data recording procedure is illustrated in Appendix B.

The clinician trained two more responses ("ships" and "cats"), which required fewer trials than the earlier stimulus items. At this point, the clinician decided to probe again, because the previous probe rate, though below criterion, was quite high. The second probe was also intermixed and showed a probe response rate of 92 percent.

To summarize, Tommy was trained in the correct production of plural /s/ with the help of six individual stimulus items. Each of the six responses was trained to a training criterion of 90 percent correct. Two structured probes were held, and the probe criterion was met on the second probe. At this point, the clinician decided to (1) initiate training on the second target behavior, and (2) shift training on the plural /s/ to the level of two word phrases.

The second target behavior was the auxiliary *is*. This feature was trained in such utterances as "boy is running," "boy is jumping," and "boy is eating." Once again, the first six of the baserated phrases were selected for the initial block of training. Consistent with the previous pattern of responses, Tommy needed modeling on the initial trials, and when it was withdrawn there were some wrong responses. Modeling was reinstated twice for the first response, once each for the next three responses. Once the evoked trials were introduced, modeling was needed for the fourth and the sixth responses. The number of training trials needed to teach the individual responses varied from 23 to 47.

An intermixed probe, conducted after six responses were trained, showed only a 33 percent correct response rate. Consequently, four more responses with the auxiliary *is* were trained. (Note: for the first target behavior, additional training was given on already trained items at a similar juncture). A second probe showed an 87 percent correct response rate on the untrained items. (Several new stimulus items were selected and added to the original probe items.) The clinician next trained two more items and probed for the third time. This probe showed a correct response rate of 95 percent. This successful probe suggested that the training on the auxiliary *is* at the level of three word phrases could be discontinued.

While the auxiliary *is* was being trained at the level of three word phrases during the first half of each session, the plural /s/ was trained at the level of two word phrases during the second half. Responses such as "two cups," "four books," and "many cats" were used. Initially, four phrases with the /s/ were trained. Modeling was needed in the beginning. However, the correct response rate showed a more rapid increase at this level. There was no need to reintroduce modeling once the evoked trials were initiated. A probe after four phrases had been trained, indicated a 76 percent response rate. Four more items were then trained. A second probe showed a response rate of 95 percent.

In the subsequent sessions, the training was initiated on the third target behavior: the preposition *on*. In each session, some time was spent in training the first two behaviors at progressively advanced levels of response complexity. When the plural /s/ met the probe criterion at the level of sentences, training on it was tentatively discontinued so that the fourth behavior — regular past tense ending with /d/ — could be trained. In this manner, all four behaviors were trained and probed at successive levels of response topography. Eventually, the behaviors met the probe criterion at the level of simple sentences evoked on discrete trials.

When the discrete trial based training was completed, the clinician probed the target behaviors in conversational speech. Tommy's correct production of the four grammatic features varied from 57 to 92 percent in conversational speech. This suggested a need to train some of the features at this level. The clinician therefore arranged conversational speech situations that provided maximum opportunities for the production of the target behaviors. Care was taken to make sure that those behaviors that were below 90 percent on the conversational probe had plenty of response opportunities. Any time the client produced one of the target responses, the clinician reinforced it. In subsequent sessions, these responses were reinforced on a variable ratio schedule of 10. Only verbal reinforcers were used. Another conversational probe indicated that no behavior was below 94 percent. At this time, the in-clinic training of the first four target behaviors — the plural /s/, the auxiliary *is*, the preposition *on*, and the regular past tense ending with /d/ — was considered complete.

If Tommy had needed training on additional grammatic features, the clinician would have continued to train those features. If not, the clinician would have assessed generalization of trained behaviors to extraclinical situations and would have instituted a maintenance program. The clinician would first have obtained a minimum of two conversational speech samples recorded at home to assess the extent of generalization. If Tommy's production of the grammatic features at home had not met the dismissal criterion of at least 90 percent correct in conversational speech, then a maintenance program would have been implemented. Most clients need such a program (see Chapter 7).

Though hypothetical, Tommy's treatment data are not unlike those often seen in real training situations. In fact, the treatment procedure, the treatment sequence, and the hypothetical results described here parallel data recorded in some of the treatment studies (Hegde, 1980; Hegde and Gierut, 1979; Hegde and McConn, 1981; Hedge, Noll, and Pecora, 1979). Figure 5–1, reproduced from a language study by Hegde, Noll, and Pecora (1979) shows the target response rates in the baseline, training, and probe sequence involving four grammatical features.

It may be noted that in Figure 5–1 each subsequent behavior has a longer baseline because of the multiple baseline design used in the study. The treatment segments in the graph show the actual response rates of a 3.9 year old boy on discrete trials. The line graphs do not show averaged response rates; they represent the child's responses on the first phrase trained in case of each of the four grammatic features. Additional stimulus items that were trained followed a similar trend although the learning was faster on many occasions.

Application of Procedure to Other Disorders

The essential procedure and the sequence just described can be applied across communicative disorders. Some modifications may have to be made, depending upon the disorder, the client, or both. More often, treatment procedures need to be modified to suit individual clients, even within the same type of communicative disorder. Such modifications can be made within the scope of the treatment principles discussed before.

In the treatment of articulation disorders, the same basic sequence can be used. The selected phonemes are baserated at the levels of single words, phrases, sentences, and conversational speech. The training is started on one or two phonemes at the single word level. Typically, target phonemes are first trained in the initial position of words. Next, the final or the medial positions of words may be

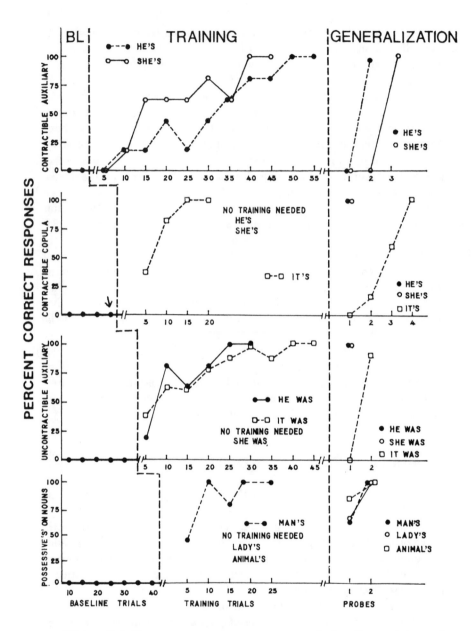

Figure 5–1. Percent correct response rates on the baseline, training and probe trials for the four grammatic features trained in a language delayed child (3.9 years). The training segments of the graph represent the actual responses given to the first stimulus item in case of each target behavior. From Hegde, M. N., Noll, M. J., and Pecora, R. (1979). A study of some factors affecting generalization of language training. *Journal of Speech and Hearing Disorder, 44;* 301–320. Reprinted with permission.

targeted for training. Each word involving the target phoneme in the initial position is trained to the training criterion of ten consecutively correct responses. Several such words are trained to such a criterion. Then an intermixed probe may be conducted to see if the trained phoneme generalizes to untrained words. If the probe criterion is met, the training may be shifted to the two word level. Also, the training may be started on the same phoneme in the medial position. At each position, treatment shifts to progressively higher levels when the probe criteria are met for the lower levels. Should treatment time permit, other phonemes or the same phoneme in other position(s) may be trained.

The treatment of stuttering also follows the same essential sequence. The target behavior in the treatment of stuttering may be an appropriate management of airflow, gentle onset of phonation, reduced speech rate, prolonged initial syllables, or other behavior. The treatment starts at the level of single words or short phrases. For example, the client is asked to reduce the syllable rate while saying single words. Each attempt on the part of the stutterer consists of a discrete trial, and the target behaviors may be scored as correct or incorrect. The training criterion here may be somewhat different from the one described before. The clinician may insist on observing a 1 percent or less dysfluency rate across two consecutive sessions. Probes can be held at this point to see if fluency can be maintained on untrained words, although these early probes can be skipped because of the extremely limited significance of fluency at the level of words or phrases. Next, the client may be asked to maintain the reduced rate of speech and fluency at the two word level. When the training criterion is met at this level, treatment may be advanced to the level of simple sentences. Gradually, the length of utterances is increased, so that eventually the client is able to maintain a reduced rate and fluency in conversational speech.

A majority of treatment techniques aimed at stuttering induce unusual patterns of speech. The stutterer may not have dysfluencies in speech, but the prosodic features may be unacceptable. The speech may be too slow or too monotonous. The normal prosodic features (socially acceptable rate and rhythm) must be shaped in gradual steps. The shaping procedure is discussed in Chapter 6.

The sequence and the basic procedures involved in the treatment of voice disorders are similar to those just described. For example, in the treatment of pitch disorders, the clinician often faces the problem of lowering or raising the vocal pitch of individual clients. The client's habitual pitch is determined through an assessment procedure. Then that pitch may be baserated at the level of single words, phrases, and sentences. The clinician might find out that the client uses a certain inappropriate pitch on 80 percent of utterances, 50 percent of the time spent in speaking, and so on. The target may be to have the client use an appropriate pitch on 90 percent of utterances or 90 percent of the time spent in speaking. The client may be given a demonstration of the desirable pitch level, and whenever that pitch is sustained on a word, or even a syllable, the clinician may reinforce it. Once again, each attempt on the part of the client is considered a trial, and the response is scored as correct or incorrect in reference to the targeted pitch.

When the client maintains the desirable pitch at the single word level with 90 percent accuracy across a set of 20 trials, treatment may be shifted to the two word level. It is probably better to skip probes at the early stages of voice therapy, also. When the training criterion is met at the two word level, more complex responses, including sentences, may be required from the client. Probes are necessary at this level of treatment. Probes sample vocal behaviors at the level of treatment, but they involve untrained phrases or sentences. When the probe criterion for conversational speech in the clinic is reached, generalization to situations outside the clinic is assessed and a maintenance program is implemented.

With suitable modifications, the same procedures and sequences can be used in the habilitation or rehabilitation of aphasic patients, those with laryngectomies, deaf individuals, and the profoundly retarded.

It must be noted that the basic sequence presented in this chapter omits certain procedures that are typically a part of most treatment programs. For example, in discussing the sequence, we have assumed that the client is able to imitate the target behaviors when they are modeled by the clinician. However, some clients may not readily imitate target responses. In such cases, the responses have to be shaped. At other stages of treatment, clients need prompting. When these procedures are used to evoke responses, they need to be faded out. These procedures are described in the next chapter. In Chapter 9, a more advanced sequence of treatment, along with suggestions on modifying planned treatment programs, will be discussed.

SUMMARY

Following an assessment, the target behaviors are selected. Baselines are then established. Baselines are response rates in the absence of treatment. Stable baselines help establish treatment effectiveness, client improvement, or both.

A two trial (one evoked, one modeled) baseline procedure was recommended. Each behavior is baserated with about 20 stimulus items. A trial is a set of events that includes stimulus manipulations, response requirement, objective recording of responses, and intertrial durations.

Baseline data are analyzed in terms of the percent correct response rate of target behaviors.

The basic treatment procedure also involves discrete trials. The target responses are modeled on the initial trials. Modeling is discontinued after five consecutively correct responses are noted. It is reinstated whenever two or more incorrect responses are observed.

A suggested tentative training criterion is ten consecutively correct evoked responses on a given training item, or 90 percent accuracy on a block of trials. A 98 percent accuracy may be used in the treatment of stuttering.

The most critical aspect of treatment is the prompt and efficient management of reinforcing and punishing consequences.

All correct and incorrect responses during baseline, treatment, and probe conditions are recorded on separate recording sheets.

The number of stimulus items to be trained depends upon the initial probe criterion. Probes assess generalized production of target responses. The initial probe criterion is 90 percent correct on untrained stimulus items, the number of which should exceed the number of trained items.

In the intermixed probe, trained and untrained items are alternated. On pure probes, only the untrained items are presented. A probe is administered after four to six items are trained. The results of either procedure are analyzed in terms of percent correct response rates.

The dismissal criterion is 90 percent or better response rate in conversational speech produced in everyday situations.

Failure to meet the initial probe criterion results in additional training on new stimulus items or already trained items.

The second and subsequent target behaviors are selected for training after the first behavior has met the initial probe criterion. Behaviors that meet the initial probe criterion may recieve additional training at more complex response topographies.

The basic sequence and the procedure can be applied across communicative disorders.

STUDY GUIDE

Answer the following questions. Use technical language. When you are not sure, reread the text and rewrite the answer. Always check your answers against the text.

1. Define baselines.
2. What is an operant level of a response?
3. Why do we need baselines?
4. What is a deteriorating baseline? Is it acceptable or not? Why?
5. Describe a baseline trial.
6. What are the four steps of the baseline procedures?
7. How do you reinforce during probes?
8. How do you determine the percent correct response rate?
9. Describe the discrete trial procedure.
10. Describe the steps involved in modeled and evoked trials.
11. What is a training trial?
12. When do you stop modeling?
13. When do you reinstate modeling?
14. What is an initial or tentative training criterion?
15. What is a probe? Why is it necessary?
16. What are the two kinds of probes?
17. What is an initial or tentative probe criterion?
18. What is a final probe criterion?
19. When do you start training on the second target behavior?
20. Define an intermixed probe. When is it used?
21. Define a pure probe. When is it used?
22. How do you reinforce during probe sessions?
23. How do you analyze probe results?
24. What are the two ways of providing additional training on already trained items?
25. Describe an initial treatment sequence with four target behaviors.
26. Illustrate with two separate disorders (language and articulation, for example) how the sequence can be applied across disorders.
27. What aspects of the treatment of stuttering and voice disorders may be different from that of articulation and language disorders?
28. Can you train more than one behavior in a training session?
29. Specify the importance of managing contingencies during training.
30. Describe the best way of reinforcing correct responses.

REFERENCES

The following studies, cited in the text, document the usefulness or effectiveness, or both, of the essential treatment program presented in this chapter. These are only a limited sampling of the available studies on treatment of communicative disorders.

Bailey, J. S., Timbers, G. D., Phillips, E. L., and Wolf, M. M. (1971). Modification of articulation errors of predelinquents by their peers. *Journal of Applied Behavior Analysis, 4,* 266–281.

Baker, R. D., and Ryan, B. P. (1971). *Programmed conditioning for articulation.* Monterey, CA: Monterey Learning Systems.

Barlow, D. H., Hayes, S. C., and Nelson, R. O. (1984). *The scientist practitioner.* New York: Pergamon.

Barrera, R. D., and Sulzer-Azaroff, B. (1983). An alternating treatment comparison of oral and total communication training programs with echolalic autistic children. *Journal of Applied Behavior Analysis, 16,* 379–394.

Bennett, C. W. (1974). Articulation training in two hearing impaired girls. *Journal of Applied Behavior Analysis, 7,* 439–445.

Blake, P., and Moss, T. (1967). The development of socialization skills in an electively mute child. *Behavior Research and Therapy. 5,* 349–356.

Brutten, G. J. (1975). Stuttering: Topography, assessment, and behavior change strategies. In J. Eisenson (Ed.), *Stuttering: A second symposium* (pp. 199–262). New York: Harper and Row.

Campbell, C., and Stremel-Campbell, K. (1982). Programming "loose training" as a strategy to facilitate language generalization. *Journal of Applied Behavior Analysis, 15,* 295–301.

Carr, E. G. (1979). Teaching autistic children to use sign language: Some research issues. *Journal of Autism and Developmental Disorders, 9,* 345–359.

Carr, E. G. (1982). *How to teach sign language to developmentally disabled children.* Lawrence, KS: H and H Enterprises.

Carr, E. G., Binkoff, J. A., Kologinsky, E., and Eddy, M. (1978). Acquisition of sign language by autistic children. I: Expressive labeling. *Journal of Applied Behavior Analysis, 11,* 489–501.

Carr, E. G., and Kologinsky, E. (1983). Acquisition of sign language by autistic children. II: Spontaneity and generalization effects. *Journal of Applied Behavior Analysis, 16,* 297–314.

Chomsky, N. (1957). *Syntactic structures.* The Hague, Netherlands: Mouton.

Chomsky, N. (1965). *Aspects of the theory of syntax.* Cambridge, MA: MIT Press.

Connell, P., and McReynolds, L. V. (1981). An experimental analysis of children's generalization during lexical learning: Comprehension or production. *Applied Psycholinguistics, 2,* 309–332.

Costello, J. M. (1977). Programmed instruction. *Journal of Speech and Hearing Disorders, 42,* 3–28.

Costello, J. M. (1980). Operant conditioning and the treatment of stuttering. In W. H. Perkins (Ed.), Strategies in stuttering therapy. *Seminars in Speech, Language and Hearing, 1,* 311–325.

Costello, J. M. (1983). Generalization across settings. In J. Miller, D. Yoder, and R. Schiefelbusch (Eds.). *Contemporary issues in language intervention* (pp. 275–297). Rockville, MD: Asha Reports No. 12.

Costello, J. M., and Onstine, J. M. (1976). The modification of multiple articulation errors based on distinctive feature theory. *Journal of Speech and Hearing Disorders, 46,* 199–215.

Duker, P. C., and Morsink, H. (1984). Acquisition and cross-setting generalization of manual signs with severely retarded individuals. *Journal of Applied Behavior Analysis, 17,* 93–103.

Elbert, M., and McReynolds, L. V. (1975). Transfer of /r/ across contexts. *Journal of Speech and Hearing Disorders, 40,* 380–387.

Faw, G. D., Reid, D. H., Schepis, M. M., Fitzgerald, J. R., and Welty, P. A. (1981). Involving institutional staff in the development and maintenance of sign langue skills with profoundly retarded persons. *Journal of Applied Behavior Analysis, 14,* 411–423.

Fitch, J. L. (1973). Voice and articulation. In B. B. Lahey (Ed.), *The modification of language behavior* (pp. 130–177). Springfield, IL: Charles C Thomas.

Flanagan, B., Goldiamond, I., and Azrin, N. H. (1958). Operant stuttering: The control of stuttering behavior through response-contingent consequences. *Journal of the Experimental Analysis of Behavior, 1,* 173–177.

Fleece, L., Gross, A., O'Brien, T., Kistner, J., Rothblum, E., and Drabman, R., (1981). Elevation of voice volume in young developmentally delayed children via an operant shaping procedure. *Journal of Applied Behavior Analysis, 14,* 351–355.

Garcia, E., and DeHaven, E. (1974). Use of operant techniques in the establishment and generalization of language: A review and analysis. *American Journal of Mental Deficiency, 79,* 169–178.

Gray, B. B. and England, G. (1969). *Stuttering and the conditioning therapies.* Monterey, CA: The Monterey Institute for Speech and Hearing.

Gray, B. B., and Ryan, B. (1971). *Programmed conditioning for language: Program book.* Monterey, CA: Monterey Learning Systems.

Gray, B. B., and Ryan, B. (1973). *A language program for the nonlanguage child.* Champagne, IL: Research Press.

Guess, D. (1969). A functional analysis of receptive language and productive speech. *Journal of Applied Behavior Analysis, 2,* 55–64.

Guess, D., and Baer, D. M. (1973a). An analysis of individual differences in generalization between receptive and productive language in retarded language. *Journal of Applied Behavior Analysis, 6,* 311–29.

Guess, D., and Baer, D. M. (1973b). Some experimental analyses of linguistic development in institutionalized retarded children. In B. B. Lahey (Ed.), *The Modification of Language Behavior* (pp. 3–60). Springfield, IL: Charles C Thomas.

Guess, D., Sailor, W., and Baer, D. M. (1978). Children with limited language. In R. L. Schiefelbusch (Ed.), *Language intervention strategies* (pp. 101–143). Baltimore: University Park Press.

Guess, D., Sailor, W., Rutherford, G., and Baer, D. M. (1968). An experimental analysis of linguistic development: The productive use of the pural morpheme. *Journal of Applied Behavior Analysis, 1,* 225–235.

Harris, S. L. (1975). Teaching language to nonverbal children with emphasis on problems of generalization. *Psychological Bulletin, 82,* 565–580.

Hegde, M. N. (1978). Fluency and fluency disorders: Their definition, measurement, and modification. *Journal of Fluency Disorders, 3,* 51–71.

Hegde, M. N. (1979). Stuttering as operant behavior. *Journal of Speech and Hearing Research, 22,* 667–669.

Hegde, M. N. (1980). An experimental-clinical analysis of grammatical and behavioral distinctions between verbal auxiliary and copula. *Journal of Speech and Hearing Research, 23,* 864–877.

Hegde, M. N. (1985). Treatment of fluency disorders: State of the art. In J. M. Costello (Ed.), *Speech disorders in adults: Recent advances* (pp. 155–188). San Diego: College-Hill Press.

Hegde, M. N., and Brutten, G. J. (1977). Reinforcing fluency in stutterers: An experimental study. *Journal of Fluency Disorders, 2,* 21–28.

Hegde, M. N., and Gierut, J. (1979). The operant training and generalization of pronouns and a verb form in a language delayed child. *Journal of Communication Disorders, 12,* 23–34.

Hegde, M. N., and McConn, J. (1981). Language training: Some data on response classes and generalization to an occupational setting. *Journal of Speech and Hearing Disorders, 46,* 353–358.

Hegde, M. N., Noll, M. J., and Pecora, R. (1979). A study of some factors affecting generalization of language training. *Journal of Speech and Hearing Disorders, 44,* 301–320.

Holland, A., and Mathews, J. (1963). Application of teaching machine concepts to speech pathology and audiology. *ASHA, 5,* 474–482.

Hurlbut, B. I., Iwata, B. A., and Green, J. D., (1982). Nonvocal language acquisition in adolescents with severe physical disabilities: Blissymbol versus iconic stimulus formats. *Journal of Applied Behavior Analysis, 15,* 241–258.

Ingham, R. J. (1984). *Stuttering and behavior therapy: Current status and experimental foundations.* San Diego: College-Hill Press.

Jackson, D. A., and Wallace, R. F. (1974). The modification and generalization of voice loudness in a fifteen-year-old retarded girl. *Journal of Applied Behavior Analysis, 7,* 461–471.

Johnston, J. M., and Johnston, G. T. (1972). Modification of consonant speech-sound articulation in young children. *Journal of Applied Behavior Analysis, 5,* 233–246.

Kazdin, A. E. (1984). *Behavior modification in applied settings* (3rd ed.). Homewood, IL: The Dorsey Press.

Koegel, R., and Rincover, A. (1977). Research on the difference between generalization and maintenance in extra-therapy responding. *Journal of Applied Behavior Analysis, 10,* 1–12.

Lane, H. L. (1964). Differential reinforcement of vocal duration. *Journal of the Experimental Analysis of Behavior, 7,* 107–115.

Lenneberg, E. H. (1967). *Biological foundations of language.* New York: Wiley.

Lovaas, I. O. (1966). A program for the establishment of speech in psychotic children. In J. K. Wing (Ed.), *Early childhood autism.* London: Pergamon.

Martin, R. R. (1968). The experimental manipulation of stuttering behaviors. In H. N. Sloane, Jr., and B. D. Macaulay (Eds.), *Operant procedures in remedial speech and language training.* Boston: Houghton Mifflin.

Martin, R. R., and Siegel, G. M. (1966). The effects of response contingent shock on stuttering. *Journal of Speech and Hearing Research, 9,* 340–352.

McDonald, J. D., and Blott, J. P. (1974). Environmental language intervention: The rationale for diagnostic training strategy through rules, context, and generalization. *Journal of Speech and Hearing Disorders. 39,* 244–256.

McNeil, D. (1970). *The acquisition of language.* New York: Harper and Row.

McReynolds, L. V. (Ed.). (1974). *Developing systematic procedures for training children's language.* Rockville, MD: ASHA Monographs No.18.

McReynolds, L. V., and Elbert, M. (1981). Generalization of correct articulation in clusters. *Applied Psycholinguistics, 2,* 119–132.

Moore, J. C., and Holbrook, A. (1971). The operant manipulation of vocal pitch in normal speakers. *Journal of Speech and Hearing Research, 14,* 283–290.

Mowrer, D. E. (1977). *Methods of modifying speech behaviors.* Columbus, OH: Charles E. Merrill.

Mowrer, D. E. (1979). *A program to establish fluent speech.* Columbus, OH: Charles E. Merrill.

Mowrer, D. E., Baker, R., and Schutz, R. (1968). *S programmed articulation control kit.* Tempe, AZ: Educational Psychological Research Associates.

Patterson, R. L., Teigen, J. R., Liberman, R. P., and Austin, N. K. (1975). Increasing speech intensity of chronic patients ("mumblers") by shaping techniques. *The Journal of Nervous and Mental Diseases, 160,* 182–187.

Remington, B., and Clark, S. (1983). Acquisition of expressive signing by autistic children: An evaluation of the relative effects of simultaneous communication and sign-alone training. *Journal of Applied Behavior Analysis, 16,* 315–328.

Rheingold, H. L., Gewirtz, J. L., and Ross, H. Q. (1959). Social conditioning of vocalizations in the infant. *Journal of Comparative and Physiological Psychology, 52,* 65–72.

Risley, T. R., and Wolf, M. M. (1967). Establishing functional speech in echolalic children. *Behavior Research and Therapy, 2,* 43–47.

Roll, D. R. (1973). Modification of nasal resonance in cleft-palate children by informative feedback. *Journal of Applied Behavior Analysis, 6,* 397–403.

Ryan, B. P. (1974). *Programmed therapy for stuttering in children and adults.* Springfield, IL: Charles C Thomas.

Sailor, W., Guess, D., Rutherford, G., and Baer, D. M. (1968). Control of tantrum behavior by operant techniques during experimental verbal training. *Journal of Applied Behavior Analysis, 1,* 237–243.

Schumaker, J. B., and Sherman, J. A. (1978). Parents as intervention agents. In R. L. Schiefelbusch (Ed.), *Language intervention strategies* (pp. 237–326). Baltimore: University Park Press.

Schumaker, J. B., and Sherman, J. A. (1970). Training generative verb usage by imitation and reinforcement procedures. *Journal of Applied Behavior Analysis, 3,* 273–287.

Schwartz, M. L., and Hawkins, R. P. (1970). Application of delayed reinforcement procedures to the behavior of an elementary school child. *Journal of Applied Behavior Analysis, 3,* 85–96.

Shames, G. H., and Florence, C. L. (1980). *Stutter-free speech: A goal for therapy.* Columbus, OH: Charles E. Merrill Co.

Shames, G. H., and Sherrick, C. E., Jr. (1963). A discussion of nonfluency and stuttering as operant behavior. *Journal of Speech and Hearing Disorders, 28,* 3–18.

Shipley, K. G., and Banis, C. (1981). *Teaching morphology developmentally.* Tucson, AZ: Communication Skill Builders.

Skinner, B. F. (1957). *Verbal Behavior.* New York: Appleton-Century-Crofts.

Todd, G. A., and Palmer, B. (1968). Social reinforcement of infant babbling. *Child Development, 39,* 591–596.

Weisberg, P. (1961). Social and nonsocial conditioning of infant vocalizations. *Child Development, 34,* 377–388.

Welch, S. (1981). Teaching generative grammar to mentally retarded children: A review and analysis of a decade of behavioral research. *Mental Retardation, 19,* 277–284.

Whaley, D. L., and Malott, R. W. (1971). *Elementary principles of behavior.* Englewood Cliffs, NJ: Prentice-Hall.

Williams, G. C., and McReynolds, L. V. (1975). The relationship between discrimination and articulation training in children with misarticulation. *Journal of Speech and Hearing Research, 18,* 401–412.

Chapter 6

Stimulus Control in Treatment

In the Chapter 5, a basic sequence of treatment, along with baseline and probe procedures that can be applied across disorders of communication was described.

In Chapter 6, the following points will be described:

- The need for some special stimulus manipulations
- Modeling and imitation
- Shaping
- Verbal instructions and prompting
- Fading

The basic sequence of a treatment program was presented in the previous chapter. It was noted that the description of the sequence did not include details of certain procedures that are used in treatment. In this chapter, some of the additional procedures that are a part of the treatment program will be described.

MODELING AND IMITATION

Showing certain pictures and asking the relevant question may be sufficient to evoke a response in some clients. However, many clients, especially young children with articulation and language problems, are not able to respond appropriately to typical stimulus conditions associated with speaking. They need not only specially prepared stimulus pictures or objects, but also modeling as a distinct form of stimulus. Therefore, the treatment sequence described in the previous chapter suggested that the clinician model the correct response on the initial trials. In fact, modeling is one of the most frequently used techniques in the treatment of communicative disorders. It is needed when responses cannot be evoked by questions and other forms of stimuli. Therefore, modeling helps teach new responses that were nonexistent in a client's repertoire. Since much of speech-language therapy is designed to bring about new responses, the importance of modeling cannot be overemphasized.

Modeling refers to a stimulus provided by the clinician, leading to a response on the part of the client. This response is called imitation. It is the clinician who models, and the client who imitates. Since modeling refers to the clinician's behavior, it can be considered a treatment (independent) variable. Imitation, on the other hand is a dependent variable. Imitation is a function of modeling and the reinforcing consequences. For these reasons, it is not appropriate to say that the technique of imitation is used in treatment.

Imitative responses can be defined as those that take the same form as their own stimuli. In other words, imitation is a behavior that duplicates its own stimulus (Winokur, 1976). When a person is imitating a model, the modeling stimulus and the imitative response take the same shape or form. The difference between the two behaviors is in a crucial temporal relation. The modeling stimulus comes first, and the imitative response follows. Thus, whether a behavior is imitative or not is judged by two criteria. An imitative behavior should (1) have the same form as the modeled stimulus and (2) follow the stimulus immediately.

The chain of modeling and imitation can be observed frequently in everyday situations. Young babies are often very good at imitation, and give an impression that they learn a lot by imitating the events in the environment. The mother claps, and the baby does the same. The mother touches her nose, and the baby gropes for his or her nose. Adults, too, learn a lot by observing other people perform various activities. A combination of verbal instructions and demonstrations play a large role in learning many complex skills. Demonstrations are nothing but modeling. When those who observe respond immediately, a chain of modeling and imitation is present.

Whether children acquire language by imitating the language responses they hear was once a subject of debate. Some psycholinguists tended to minimize the importance of imitation in the language acquisition process (Dale, 1976; Owens, 1984). Other scientists thought that although imitation would not account for everything the child learned to say, it did play an important role (McLaughlin and Cullinan 1981; Winokur, 1976). If children did not imitate speech sounds, syllables, and words, then the learning process would probably be prolonged. Individual syllables and words would then have to be shaped. Indeed, that is what a clinician does when a child has not acquired language and does not readily imitate speech. The child's tendency to imitate speech provides a foundation on which to build a more complex set of verbal skills.

From a clinical standpoint, whether modeling and imitation are involved in the normal language acquisition is not as important as it may seem. If there is controlled clinical research showing that modeling and imitation are useful techniques, they can be used in treatment regardless of how language is "normally" acquired. There is very little experimental evidence to support the widely held belief that clinical treatment must follow the processes thought to be a part of normal acquisition of communicative behaviors. Certain processes observed in normal acquisition may not be necessary for clinical treatment. For example, behaviors normally mastered earlier need not necessarily be taught before those that are mastered later (Capelli, 1985; De Cesari, 1985; Hegde, 1980). On the other hand, certain other processes such as modeling that may not play a major role in normal acquisition process may have to be used in treatment sessions.

There is plenty of clinical evidence on the usefulness of modeling in the treatment of speech, language, voice, and fluency disorders (Guess and Baer, 1973b; Guess, Sailor, and Baer, 1978; Harris, 1975; Hegde, 1980; Hegde, Noll, and Pecora, 1979; McLaughlin and Cullinan, 1981; Welch, 1981). In the early part of treatment, modeling is often essential, although there is no guarantee that the client will be able to imitate the correct response when the clinician models it. When the client does not imitate at all, then the imitative behaviors should be shaped in gradual steps before nonimitative responses can be taught. The shaping procedure will be described later in the chapter. When the client can imitate the target behaviors, the initial treatment phase can be relatively easy and short.

When to Model

Modeling is considered a special stimulus condition, and therefore it is needed whenever the typical stimuli such as questions and actual events do not evoke target behaviors. A language disordered child, for example, may not use the plural inflection when questioned about plural objects and events. A nonverbal child may not name objects or pictures when they are presented. It is probably of no use telling a child not to distort the /s/ in speech. When a stuttering client is told to "slow down," the rate may not be reduced. Modeling is needed in situations such as these. In most cases, the clinician has to produce the required behavior in the manner expected of the client.

The need for modeling is probably the greatest in the initial phase of treatment. This is the time when the client has no idea what the clinician wants. Typically, clinicians model consistently on the initial trials until an objective criterion, such as five consecutively correct imitated responses, is met. In subsequent stages of treatment, modeling is needed whenever the evoked procedure fails on consecutive trials. In this sense, modeling is a procedure that guards against repeated failures by the client. A few wrong responses on the evoked trials should result in the reinstatement of modeling. Consequently, correct (imitated) responses may once again be likely. This will prevent a potential extinction schedule or excessive punishment because of wrong responses on evoked trials.

Modeling may also be needed every time the treatment is shifted to a new phase or level. Although phases of treatment can and often do vary across individuals and disorders, some common phases are relatively constant. Typically, treatment is started at the level of single words or syllables and progresses through the levels of phrases, sentences, and conversational speech. This is true regardless of the diagnostic category and the age of the client. Whether it is the production of a phoneme, a grammatic morpheme, a gentle phonatory onset, or a certain vocal pitch, clients are asked to learn new skills in levels of increasing response complexity.

The clinician may often find out that when a new phase of treatment is introduced, the correct response rate is lower than that recorded in the phase just completed. A child who has achieved 90 percent correct production of /s/ in the initial position of words may drop down to 30 percent correct when moved to the two word level. A stutterer who can achieve gentle phonatory onset at the level of single words with 99 percent accuracy may revert to abrupt onset when moved to phrases or sentences. Therefore, at each of these new phases of treatment, modeling may be necessary.

The need for modeling in the subsequent phases of treatment should not be as great as in the initial phases. There should be a progressive reduction in the amount of modeling used across treatment phases. Marked need for modeling in the latter phases of treatment suggests that the evoked trials are not as effective as they should be. In the very final stages of treatment, such as those involving conversational speech in and outside the clinic, the need for modeling should be occasional, if at all. Excessive need for modeling in the final phases of treatment means that the target behavior has not been brought under its usual stimulus control. It may also mean that the client was moved too fast from phase to phase, resulting in insufficient amount of treatment at each phase.

How to Model

As described in the previous chapter, the clinician models the response the way the client is expected to produce it. If, on the evoked trials, questions are used to evoke responses, then on the modeled trials, modeling is given only after the relevant question is asked. If the response is modeled in the absence of the question, it becomes difficult to move on to the evoked trials, because on these trials, what evokes a response is the question. There is no continuity between modeled and evoked trials when questions are a part of only the evoked trials. Such interruptions in the treatment process can disrupt the correct response rate. Therefore, the question to be used in evoking the response should precede the modeled response. For example, if the clinician plans to ask "what is the boy doing?" to evoke a *verb* + *ing*, then on the modeled trial, the question is asked first and immediately, "Say, the boy is running" is added (Hegde et al., 1979).

In the treatment of language disorders, the specific target response or responses may be a part of an utterance that contains nontarget responses. The example just given is a case in point. The target response being taught may be just the *ing*; the child may be able to produce the main verb. Or, the target response may be *is* and *ing* (the auxiliary and the present progressive). In either case, the sentence used on the training trials contains nontarget responses. In such situations, a vocal emphasis on the target responses can be helpful. When the clinician increases the vocal intensity on the specific target responses ("say the boy *is* run*ning*"), the client may be more likely to imitate those targets. Sometimes, this procedure is described as a prompt, but prompts can be a part of modeling. There are other ways in which a response can be prompted, and those will be described later in this chapter.

Regardless of the disorder being treated, modeling is useful. In the treatment of stuttering, the clinician may model the reduced rate of speaking, gentle onset of phonation, or prolongation of the initial syllable of words. Even with adult speakers, it is often not sufficient to tell them that they should reduce the rate of speech or that they should prolong the initial syllable of words. The clinician will have to demonstrate a rate that is judged to be adequate to eliminate stutterings. Often, the rate at which stutterings decrease in a given client must be determined empirically. In other words, a suitable rate must be found for each client through informal experimentation.

In the rate control treatment of stuttering, it is very useful if the clinician also speaks at a noticeably slower rate. In this case, a certain rate is modeled and expected to be imitated, but what is said by the clinician is not imitated. If the questions are asked in a hurry, or at a very fast rate, it may be difficult for the client to answer at a relatively slow rate. A question asked at a slower rate has a better chance of being answered at a slower rate than the one asked at a faster rate.

Modeling is equally necessary in the treatment of voice disorders. In treating a vocal intensity disorder, for example, the clinician may have to model the louder or softer level that is being targeted for a given client. Modeling techniques may be equally necessary in the treatment of resonance disorders. Reduced or increased nasality on appropriate target sounds (and words) may have to be modeled before the client can imitatively produce responses with appropriate resonance.

Correct production of speech sounds in the treatment of articulation is almost invariably modeled, even though clients are not often able to imitate the sounds in the initial stages of treatment (Fitch, 1973; Mowrer and Case, 1982; Williams and McReynolds, 1975). Modeling in the treatment of articulation can take different forms. Most modeled responses have what the clinician considers to be the appropriate acoustic (audible) properties of the target sounds. This is the typical "say *sun*" variety of modeling. But modeling can also be nonacoustic, and purely topographic. This type of modeling involves a demonstration of the "correct placement" of articulators in the production of target phonemes. The clinician might silently demonstrate the position of the tongue for the production of /l/, or the relationship between the upper dental arch and the lower lip in the production of /f/. A distorted /s/ can sometimes be modified by modeling a very soft /s/ produced with minimum articulatory effort.

Reinforcing Imitative Behaviors

Correctly imitated behaviors are immediately reinforced by the clinician. Sometimes, the client may not be able to imitate the response fully. A question then arises as to whether the client should be reinforced or not. For example, the clinician might model the correct production of an /s/ in the initial position of words, but the child's response may not be an accurate imitation. Or, the clinician might model a word response in teaching a core vocabulary to a nonverbal child, but the child's response might at best be a partial imitation. Technically, imitative behaviors must resemble the modeled stimulus very closely. If not, they are not imitative behaviors, and therefore they may not be reinforced.

In clinical practice, insistence upon technically defined imitative behaviors can create problems in the initial stages of treatment. The client may just not be able to imitate the modeled response fully, and therefore may never receive reinforcers. To avoid this situation, clinicians usually reinforce a response if it shows some improvement, or a sign of movement in the right direction. The clinician usually judges whether the attempted imitation is better than the responses typically given by the client on the baseline trials. If it is, the response may be accepted as imitative, and be reinforced accordingly.

When less than full imitations are accepted, the clinician should gradually raise the criterion of performance accuracy in order to receive reinforcers. In other words, what was acceptable on the initial trials may not be acceptable on subsequent trials. Progressively better imitations must be required to earn reinforcers. Eventually, the client responses should match the modeled stimulus as fully as possible.

The procedure in which less than desirable responses are accepted initially, and the criterion of performance is raised gradually as the client's level of mastery increases is known as shaping or successive approximations. The procedure is not limited to modeling-imitation sequences, and it is described later in the chapter.

Discriminative Modeling

Some clients may benefit from a type of modeling in which the correct and the incorrect responses are modeled consecutively, asking the client to imitate the correct form. The client's faulty production of a speech sound, the inappropriate pitch, or the habitual rate of speech can be occasionally modeled and contrasted with the desirable responses in each case. It is preferable to model first the inappropriate form and then the appropriate form of the target response. This way, the client can be expected to imitate the correct form as soon as it is modeled.

Whether the client should occasionally imitate the wrong response whose frequency is already reduced is a question that cannot be answered firmly. At one time, clients were asked to repeatedly practice their error response under the name of negative practice. The clinician in this case may model the client's wrong responses. Actually, there is very little experimental support for this method. It is probably not very useful to have the client practice the wrong responses. Once in a while, though, some clients seem to get a better "feel" for the correct response if they produce their own wrong responses modeled by the clinician. This may be useful when done only occasionally.

It is possible that the modeling of both the correct and incorrect responses (and the subsequent imitation of both by the client) encourages discrimination between correct and incorrect responses. What is referred to here is the discriminated rates of responses, not auditory or any other form of perceptual discrimination. By periodically punishing the imitated wrong response and immediately reinforcing the correct response, the clinician may strengthen the correct form while weakening the incorrect one. It must be noted that there is a need to experimentally evaluate discriminative modeling before it can be used routinely.

Fading or Discontinuation of Modeling

As noted earlier, modeling is an additional stimulus provided by the clinician in order to gain control over the client's response. Explicit modeling is typically not a natural stimulus variable. Therefore, modeling must be used only when necessary, and it must be discontinued as soon as possible. However, it is always possible that when modeling is discontinued, the client may not give the correct response. Because of this, the clinician should give some thought to the manner in which modeling is discontinued.

Modeling can either be withdrawn all at once, or faded in gradual steps. In the former procedure, the clinician simply stops modeling as soon as a criterion of imitative responses has been met. The evoked trial procedure is then introduced. In the other procedure, modeling is not withdrawn abruptly, but faded gradually. In fading the modeled stimulus control, the clinician progressively reduces the length of the modeled utterance. The longer the modeled utterance, the greater the steps involved in fading it. Obviously, this procedure is most effective when the modeled utterance contains multiple words. There is a better chance that the correct response rate will be maintained when the modeled stimulus is faded than when it is withdrawn.

In fading the modeled stimulus, the clinician first drops the last word of the utterance with a rising intonational pattern. Sometimes, what is dropped may be a morphologic component of the last word. The resulting modeled utterance may sound like a sentence completion task. For example, suppose that a child is being trained in the production of the present progressive (*ing*). The clinician models the sentence "the boy is running," and the client meets the initial criterion of five consecutively correct imitated responses. Assume that whenever modeling is discontinued, the child does not maintain the correct response. This suggests that the behavior is under the control of the modeled stimulus, and this control must be faded, not abruptly eliminated.

In this case, the clinician can model the response without the *ing*. After having asked the relevant question, the clinician models "Tommy, say, The boy is run...," with a rising intonational pattern, which resembles a question, and suggests that the utterance is not complete. If the response is only "running" and is not acceptable, then the client can be instructed to "start with *the boy*." If the client is able to maintain the correct response rate, the clincian can drop the word *run*. The modeled stimulus would then be "Tommy, say, The boy is..." In subsequent steps the words *is*, *boy*, and *the* would be dropped one at a time. Eventually, only the question is asked, and time is allowed for the response to occur.

The procedure of fading the modeled stimulus control can also be called partial modeling. In turn, the partial modeling can also be considered verbal prompts. In the example above, the verbal prompts (partial models) are parts of an answer supplied by the clinician who also asked the question. However, some forms of prompts do not contain any part or parts of the response expected of the client, and therefore they are unlike partial models. A variety of prompts is used in shaping a new response, and they will be described in a later section.

SHAPING

As noted in the previous section, modeling is a technique that helps the clinician teach a new response as long as the client can imitate it, even imperfectly. However, some clients cannot imitate a modeled stimulus unless some other special procedures are used. Such clients cannot be taught new behaviors with the straightforward modeling-imitation-reinforcement sequence. Also, certain target behaviors can be very complex, and unless they are simplified, the client may not be able to learn them. Complex responses are simplified by breaking them into smaller components. In sequential steps, the learned components are put together to achieve the final, complex, integrated, behavior.

When a client cannot imitate a response that is not in his or her repertoire, or when the response is complex and needs to be broken into smaller components, or both, the clinician can use the shaping procedure. The procedure is also known as successive approximation (Kazdin, 1984; Sundel and Sundel, 1975; Whaley and Malott, 1971). It has been used widely in the treatment of speech and language disorders. Essentially, shaping is the technique designed to bring about new behaviors. The straightforward positive reinforcement technique can increase responses that already exist in the client's repertoire, but it cannot create new behaviors unless combined with modeling and shaping. From a clinical standpoint, new behaviors have to be created in many clients who are nonverbal, who cannot imitate the target behaviors, or who find the final target behavior (meaningful communicative behaviors) too complex to master in total.

How to Shape a Response

Shaping, like any other treatment procedure, starts with the selection and definition of a target behavior according to the procedures described in Chapter 3. Once the target behavior has been selected, the clinician will baserate the response. When both the evoked and modeled trials are used in baselining the behavior, the clinician would know whether the client can imitate the responses or not. If the rate of imitative behavior is close to zero, then there is probably a need for shaping. Also, the need for shaping may become evident at any stage of treatment. When the treatment moves to a more complex level, the client may not be able to imitate the more complex responses.

As was noted in earlier chapters, a final or dismissal criterion is the production of clinically taught behaviors in conversational speech emitted in everyday situations. It means that almost invariably, the final target behavior is too complex to be attempted in the initial treatment phases. Therefore, the treatment almost always starts at a certain lower level at which the client can perform the required response with the help of modeling. Consequently, the shaping procedure is integral to most treatment programs. Therefore, the specific steps of the shaping procedure described below apply to most treatment programs.

Step 1: Describe the Terminal Response. In the shaping procedure, the final target is called the terminal response. For example, with a nonverbal child, a terminal target might be the production of selected words in conversational speech emitted in the child's home and other situations. The words to be taught are specified. However, the child is not able to imitate the words. Also, the treatment is not started at the conversational speech level. Therefore, we need to identify a starting point.

Step 2: Describe the Initial Response. The initial response must fulfill two basic criteria: (1) the client should at least be able to imitate it, and (2) it must bear a relation to the terminal response. Let us say that the first target word to be taught to the nonverbal child is "Mommy." The initial response in this case may be putting the upper and lower lips together so that the initial articulatory posture for the production of /m/ is achieved. The child can probably imitate it with the help of some additional procedures we will describe shortly. The articulatory posture bears a systematic relation to the response "Mommy."

Step 3: Describe the Intermediate Responses. The intermediate responses bridge the gap between the initial and the terminal responses. These responses form a chain so that when trained systematically and in sequence, the end result is the production of the terminal response. It is often difficult to specify all of the intermediate responses needed to achieve a terminal response. In order to teach the same response, one client may need more intermediate responses than another client. The target response must be broken into more and smaller components with a client who needs to be trained with additional intermediate responses. Therefore, the clinician must be able to identify smaller components of terminal responses.

In the example just given, some of the intermediate responses may include the following: vocalization while the lips are in the articulatory posture for the production of /m/, which might result in a nasal resonance; opening the mouth when this vocal response is still being made; closing the mouth again; and opening the mouth while adding an /i/ sound. These intermediate responses should be taught in that order. The resulting response will be an approximation of "Mommy," which needs to be "put together" and practiced again.

Step 4: Model the Specific Response under Training. The specific response under training may be the initial, the terminal, or one of the intermediate responses. Each response is modeled in its initial stage of training. The criteria for modeling, evoking, and reintroducing modeling can be the same as described before (Chapter 5). The nonvocal (or nonverbal) responses should be modeled, all the same. In our example, the clinician would model the articulatory posture for the initial /m/.

Step 5: Use Manual Guidance When Necessary. When the child does not imitate the modeled response, manual guidance is needed. The clinician may have to first model the needed response, and immediately manually guide the response. In teaching the initial articulatory response for the production of /m/, the clinician models the posture and then manually "shapes" the client's lips a few times. In teaching appropriate pointing responses, a clinician may say "show me the cup" and immediately take the client's hand and point to the appropriate picture. This is another example of manual guidance. It is probably more frequently used with nonverbal and retarded clients. It is needed whenever the child fails to imitate the response.

Step 6: Reinforce the Correct Responses. Correctly imitated responses are immediately reinforced. Usually, imitated responses are reinforced on a continuous basis. Subsequently, when the responses are evoked, an intermittent schedule of reinforcement is used. However, any of the intermediate responses should not be excessively reinforced. If this were to happen, it would be difficult to move on to the next response in the hierarchy. Sometimes clinicians talk about clients who "get stuck" or "perseverate" during treatment. This may be a consequences of overly reinforcing an intermediate response in a shaping program.

As soon as an initial or an intermediate response shows a consistent increase over the level observed in the beginning, the clinician must move on to the next response. In this way, the sequence of responses is taught as quickly as possible. The terminal response, however, needs to be strengthened so that it is maintained. Therefore, it should receive more training than the initial and the intermediate responses. The training and probe criteria for the terminal response are the same as those discussed in Chapter 5.

The six steps described here can make it possible to train most new responses. Shaping is a valuable tool in the treatment of autistic and mentally retarded children who may not readily imitate target behaviors. In teaching syntactical structures, shaping can be useful with any client. For example, a target behavior such as "the boy is running" may not be fully imitated by the client. The clinician then asks the client to imitate "the boy" and subsequently "is running," and finally "the boy is running."

The rehabilitation of the aphasic patient typically requires the shaping procedure. The more severe the aphasic condition, the greater the need for the shaping procedure. In many cases, manual guidance, extensive prompts, frequent modeling, and simple response topographies that are changed in small increments are all a part of most treatment programs designed for severe aphasic patients.

In the treatment of articulation disorders, the terminal response is usually the production of target sounds in conversational speech in extraclinical situations. This target is achieved in small steps starting with the production of a given sound in "isolation," syllables, words, phrases, and sentences. When the client cannot make the sound in isolation, the clinician might ask the child to simply move an articulator in a certain direction. The child trying to learn the production of /l/, for example, may be asked to lift the tip of the tongue and touch the alveolar ridge. When this response is performed reliably, the clinician might ask the child to vocalize while the tongue tip is in contact with the alveolar ridge. Next, the child might be asked to release the air stream by lowering the tongue tip. The resulting sound would resemble an /l/. Additional intermediate responses would be trained at the level of syllables, words, phrases, and sentences.

The sequence of responses involved in the treatment of voice disorders is similar to that just described. A client with excessive nasality may be asked to say /a/ without nasal resonance (initial response). Nonnasal productions of /a/ are immediately reinforced. When the client has done this a few times, the /a/ may be shaped into a simple word such as *all*. Additional syllables and words may be added to expand the utterance length, reinforcing each of the intermediate responses until they are all produced consistently.

Shaping plays a major role in the treatment of fluency disorders. In achieving targets such as a reduced speech rate, gentle onset of phonation, prolongation of syllables of words, or airstream management, the treatment starts at a simple level of response topography. The initial response is usually one or two words spoken at a time while the new skills are practiced. Intermediate responses include progressively longer utterances produced with the specific target topography. Each increment in the length of an utterance might constitute an intermediate response in the overall treatment program.

In the treatment of adult stutterers, there is a different kind of need for the shaping procedure. Many of the target responses specified here result in a pattern of speech that is not socially acceptable. The client whose speech rate is dramatically reduced does not "sound" normal, even though the speech is devoid of most forms of stuttering. Speech is similarly altered when clients are taught to prolong the initial syllables of words, to initiate each sound in a very gentle manner, or manage the breathing explicitly for the purposes of fluency. Under each of these treatment targets, the resulting speech will not have some aspects of normal prosody. Consequently, in the final phases of treatment, normal prosodic features must be shaped. A more natural-sounding rate, subtle management of the airstream during speech production, and phonatory onset that does not draw social attention must be shaped in gradual steps. Thus, in the treatment of stuttering, shaping is needed first to reduce dysfluencies, and then to shape normal prosodic features.

In case of young stuttering children, a straightforward technique of reinforcing fluent utterances can be effective (Costello, 1980). In this technique, a child stutterer is not taught a particular skill such as gentle phonatory onset. Even then, the treatment starts with an initial response (such as single word utterances) which is reinforced when spoken fluently. Intermediate responses once again include utterances of increased lengths. The terminal response is conversational speech produced fluently in everyday situations. Because this type of treatment does not alter the pattern of speech, there is no need to shape the prosodic features of speech.

INSTRUCTIONS AND PROMPTS

In spite of the fact that our profession is mostly concerned with speech and language, the role of verbal instructions and prompts remains one of the least researched techniques of behavior change. Yet, in everyday situations, verbal instructions (and prompts, to a lesser extent) play a major role in controlling human behavior. Many skills, ranging from washing a dish, learning the alphabet, and playing a piano to ballet dancing, are taught through verbal instructions combined with modeling. The pupil listens to the instructions, watches demonstrations, and then tries to duplicate the action. Many "do it like this" demonstrations are a combination of modeling and verbal instructions. After some learning has taken place, prompts ("hints") can increase the probability of the skill being performed. Prompts are then removed in gradual steps so that responses are maintained without these additional stimuli.

Instructions are verbal stimuli that gain control over another person's actions. They illustrate a special kind of stimulus control of behavior. For the most part, subhuman behaviors are under the control of chemical and physical stimuli. Many human behaviors, too, are under the control of those kinds of stimuli. However, one distinct aspect of human behavior is the verbal stimulus control, which makes the process of learning adaptive as well as creative behaviors relatively efficient. Instructions combined with modeling spare the learner of the tedious, slow workings of natural contingencies. Instead of fumbling through the sequence of actions, making many mistakes, and thus learning the hard way, one can listen, watch, perform, and learn new skills with fewer mistakes and in less time.

Although modeling is the actual demonstration of a response, it is mostly preceded or accompanied by verbal instructions. Before a tongue placement for the correct production of a speech sound is modeled, the sequence of actions involved is usually described. Descriptions of the following kind may be given frequently: "See the tip of my tongue? I am going to make it real small like this. Then I am going to lift it up. See? Then the tip of of my tongue is going to touch this part of my mouth. Did you see that? You think you can do it?" Also, just before modeling, "do as I do" types of instructions are given. Without these additional stimuli, the client may or may not imitate the modeled response. The initial treatment sequence is often described as modeling-imitation-reinforcement, but it is better described as instructions-modeling-imitation-reinforcement. Instructions are useful in the initial as well as subsequent phases of treatment. Instructions given during the latter stages of treatment may be more complex.

With some clients who seem to learn the target behaviors fast, the clinician need not model very frequently. In the treatment of such clients, instructions may play an even more important role. Specific instructions, a minimum amount of modeling, and reinforcement contingencies may constitute an effective treatment program for such clients.

Much research work regarding the effects of instructions on target behaviors remains to be done. It must be recognized that instructions alone may not be effective in many cases. However, when combined with modeling, shaping, and contingent consequences, instructions can be very useful.

Prompts

Prompts are also special stimuli that increase the probability of evoking responses (Kazdin, 1984). Prompts are like "hints" of everyday life. A question is asked, and when the response is not forthcoming readily, an additional stimulus is given. This stimulus may draw the response from an unsure person.

Prompts can be verbal or nonverbal. Some verbal prompts are similar to partial modeling. After having asked the question "what is the boy doing?" the clinician might say "the boy is..." and wait for an answer. This partial modeling works like a prompt. The chances of the client saying "the boy is *running*" may be enhanced by the prompt. As suggested in an earlier section, this type of prompt is an excellent way of fading the stimulus control exerted by modeling. In gradual steps, more of the modeled response is omitted. It may be noted that this type of prompt contains parts of the answer or the target behavior under training.

A study has shown that vocal emphasis can be a prompt (Risley and Reynolds, 1970). In teaching various grammatical features, the clinician might place an extra emphasis on the target behavior under training. This is done on the modeled trials. For example, the clinician might ask, "say, the boy is runn*ing*" while giving an extra vocal emphasis on the *ing*.

There are verbal prompts that need not contain any part of the response expected. Some times, the clinician might ask "what do you say?" or "do you remember?" after having asked the question designed to evoke the answer. Such promptings may lead to correct responses in some cases.

Nonverbal or physical prompts are various gestures and motor behaviors that suggest the target behavior to the client. After having asked the same question "what is the boy doing?" the clinician might gesture motion. The client then might immediately say "running." While training the correct production of /l/ in the initial position of words, the clinician might show the picture of an /l/ word and ask the client to name it. Before the client makes an attempt, the clinician might demonstrate the tongue-tip position needed for the production of /l/. The clinician does not produce the sound or the word itself. Such physical prompts are frequently given once the client has shown that he or she can imitate the response modeled by the clinician.

In the treatment of fluency and voice disorders, certain gestures can be used to prompt the target behaviors. If the treatment target is a lower pitch level, the clinician can hand-gesture at a relatively low level during conversational speech. A gesture at a higher level can be used to signal the fact that the client's pitch is too high. While reducing a stutterer's speech rate, the clinician can show a slower hand movement as a prompt for reduced speech rate.

Prompts should not be confused with manual guidance. In manual guidance, the required response is physically shaped by the clinician. When the clinician moves the lips of the client, or takes the client's hand and makes it point to the appropriate picture, the entire response is being physically guided. Prompts, on the other hand, contain at best only a part of the response required of the client, and there is no physical contact with the client. Many physical prompts may not contain any part of the target response at all.

By and large, the need for prompts should be minimal. A few prompts should lead to evoked trials so that there is no need for either modeling or prompts. If the clinician must prompt constantly, it means that more modeled trials were needed.

FADING

It is clear that the treatment of communicative disorders involves extensive manipulation of stimulus conditions. The fact that a client seeks clinical services means that perhaps natural stimuli encountered in everyday situations have not entered into a contingency. In other words, a normally speaking person would find a "lot of things to talk about," but a language delayed child may not. Technically speaking, objects and events surrounding the child have not acquired the discriminative stimulus value (see Chapter 7). Therefore, the clinician arranges a variety of special stimulus conditions, including pictures, modeling, instructions, manual guidance, and prompts so that the client will learn to respond verbally and appropriately to stimulus conditions encountered in everyday life.

It is also clear that the special stimulus conditions manipulated by the clinician, by definition, are not a typical part of the client's environment. The parents of a language handicapped child do not systematically arrange pictorial stimuli, followed by explicit questions, modeling, prompting, and so on. Therefore, even when correct responses are reliably given in treatment sessions, the client may fail to respond appropriately in everyday situations that lack the special stimulus support. This means that the two situations are discriminated. The home situation is different from the clinical situation. Consequently, the responses produced in the clinic may not be produced at home.

The client can respond reliably in extraclinical situations when the clinical and nonclinical situations are not discriminated. That is, if the two situations are similar in terms of stimuli and consequences, then the responses learned in one situation may be produced in the other. Since the special stimulus conditions associated with treatment create a difference between clinical and nonclinical situations, steps should be taken to minimize or eliminate this difference. The technique designed to make the treatment conditions more like everyday situations is known as fading (Whaley and Malott, 1971).

Fading can be defined as a technique in which the special stimulus control of target behaviors created and exerted by the clinician is reduced in gradual steps. While the same responses are evoked, the special stimuli are gradually withdrawn. Various apsects of fading have been discussed in the context of modeling. The procedure will be summarized here.

It has been pointed out before that partial modeling is a way to fade modeling. At other times, a modeled stimulus can be faded in terms of its acoustic properties. Initially, the clinician models the response with an appropriate level of vocal intensity. As soon as the client begins to imitate the reponse reliably, the clinician can reduce the vocal intensity of modeling. The clinician would model in a softer and softer voice on successive trials until the voice is completely faded out.

Sometimes, when the voice is faded out, the client may stop responding correctly. In such situations, additional fading steps can be introduced. The clinician can just "mouth" the target response without vocalization. These articulatory movements can also be faded. On successive trials, fewer and fewer movements can be modeled. Or, the movements can be less and less conspicuous on succeeding trials.

Pictures used on discrete treatment trials can also be faded. The picture is initially placed right in front of the client. The clinician can begin to move it around on the table so that eventually it is no longer in front of the client. Finally, the picture can be removed from the client's sight.

Manual guidance is faded similarly. The extent of guidance can be reduced gradually. To begin with, the clinician may take the child's hand and point to the correct picture while making a "show me..." type of request. Soon, the hand may be moved close to the relevant picture, and the child is allowed to actually touch it. Then, only the initial movement of the hand may be guided by the clinician. Next, a gentle touch on the hand may be sufficient to initiate the response. In this manner, the entire manual guidance can be faded out, so that the correct pointing response is given as soon as the request is made by the clinician.

Nonverbal prompts can be faded very much like manual guidance. The hand gestures suggesting a certain pitch level or speech rate can be made less and less conspicuous. The time duration for which the gesture is held can also be reduced gradually until it is eliminated. The position or movement of articulators used to prompt the correct production of speech sounds can be similarly faded.

Verbal prompts can be faded the way modeling is faded. Prompts are faded in terms of either acoustic properties or response topographies. In the former procedure, the vocal intensity of the prompt is reduced until it is no longer heard. In the latter procedure, the number of response components modeled is reduced in gradual steps.

Fading Other Kinds of Stimulus Control

As noted before, fading is critical from the standpoint of generalization and maintenance. The potential for generalization is enhanced when modeling, prompts, and other such stimulus manipulations are faded. However, there are still other kinds of special stimuli associated with treatment, and they too must be faded. The entire physical setup of treatment, and the clinician who provides the treatment, can become special discriminative stimuli for target responses. Natural settings and audiences other than the clinician may lead to discrimination rather than generalization. In many cases, therefore, the stimulus control exerted by the physical setup and the clinician must also be faded out. Fading these and other kinds of stimuli to enhance generalization and maintenance is described in the next chapter.

SUMMARY

Many clients need special stimuli without which the target responses are not produced at all. A significant part of treatment is to create stimulus control for nonexistent communicative behaviors.

Modeling is the clinician's response that the client imitates. The clinician produces the target behavior and asks the client to reproduce it. It is a very frequently used technique.

Imitation is the client response that reproduces its own stimulus. Clinically, approximations of stimuli are often accepted and reinforced.

Shaping is a technique designed to teach nonexistent target behaviors. In this procedure, a terminal target behavior is broken down into an initial response and several intermediate responses. All responses are modeled and reinforced. In successive stages, more complex topographies are trained.

Manual guidance is a procedure in which the response is physically shaped or directed by the clinician.

Prompts and instructions are also important aspects of special stimulus control used in treatment. Verbal instructions are often accompanied by demonstrations. Prompts can be verbal or nonverbal.

Special stimulus control procedures such as modeling, prompts, manual guidance and instructions must be faded in gradual steps. If not, the target behaviors may not generalize to natural environments.

STUDY GUIDE

Answer the following questions in technical language. Verify your answers against the text. Rewrite inadequate answers.

1. What is stimulus control?
2. Define modeling and imitation.
3. What kind of variables are modeling and imitation (dependent/ independent)?
4. State the two criteria for judging whether a response is imitative.
5. Do you think the modeling-imitation-reinforcement sequence should not be used in clinical language training if it is demon-

strated that children do not normally learn language in that manner?

6. What kinds of evidence are required to decide whether a modeling-imitation-reinforcement sequence should or should not be used clinically?
7. State the need for modeling.
8. When do you model?
9. Do you require perfect stimulus-response matching for reinforcement in the initial stages of training? Justify your answer.
10. Define discriminative modeling.
11. What are the two methods of discontinuing modeling?
12. What is a partial modeling?
13. Define shaping.
14. When do you need to use shaping?
15. What is another name for shaping?
16. Describe the six steps of shaping.
17. What are the two kinds of shaping needed in some stuttering treatment programs?
18. Define verbal instructions.
19. Describe the importance of verbal instructions.
20. Describe a prompt.
21. Distinguish between verbal and nonverbal prompts. Give examples.
22. As described in the text, what is a vocal emphasis?
23. Describe fading.
24. Specify the need for fading.
25. What is "fading in terms of acoustic properties"?
26. Why is fading helpful for generalization?
27. What is manual guidance?
28. What are all the variables that need to be faded out?

REFERENCES

Capelli, R. (1985). *An experimental analysis of morphologic acquisition.* Unpublished master's thesis, California State University, Fresno.

Costello, J. M. (1980). Operant conditioning and the treatment of stuttering. In W. H. Perkins (Ed.), Strategies in stuttering therapy. *Seminars in Speech, Language and Hearing, 1,* 311–325. New York: Thieme-Stratton.

De Cesari, R. (1985). *Experimental training of grammatic morphemes: Effects on the order of acquisition.* Unpublished master's thesis, California State University, Fresno.

Dale, P. S. (1976). *Language development: Structure and function* (2nd ed.). New York: Holt, Rinehart and Winston.

Fitch, J. L. (1973). Voice and articulation. In B. B. Lahey (Ed.), *The modification of language behavior* (pp. 130–177). Springfield, IL: Charles C Thomas.

Guess, D. and Baer, D. M. (1973). Some experimental analyses of linguistic development in institutionalized retarded children. In B. B. Lahey (Ed.), *The modification of language behavior* (pp. 3–60). Springfield, IL: Charles C Thomas.

Guess, D., Sailor, W., and Baer, D. M. (1978). Children with limited language. In R. L. Schiefelbusch (Ed.), *Language intervention strategies* (pp. 101–143). Baltimore: University Park Press.

Harris, S. L. (1975). Teaching language to nonverbal children with emphasis on problems of generalization. *Psychological Bulletin, 82*, 565–580.

Hegde, M. N. (1980). An experimental-clinical analysis of grammatical and behavioral distinctions between verbal auxiliary and copula. *Journal of Speech and Hearing Research, 23*, 864–877.

Hegde, M. N., Noll, M. J., and Pecora, R. (1979). A study of some factors affecting generalization of language training. *Journal of Speech and Hearing Disorders, 44*, 301–320.

Kazdin, A. E. (1984). *Behavior modification in applied settings* (3rd Ed.). Homewood, IL: Dorsey Press.

McLaughlin, S. F., and Cullinan, W. (1981). An empirical perspective on language development and language training. In N. J. Lass (Ed.), *Speech and Language: Advances in basic research and practice* (Vol. 5) (pp. 249–310). New York: Academic Press.

Mowrer, D. E., and Case, J. L. (1982). *Clinical management of speech disorders*. Rockville, MD: Aspen Publications.

Owens, R. E. (1984). *Language development: An introduction*. Columbus, OH: Charles E. Merrill.

Sundel, M., and Sundel, S. S. (1975). *Behavior modification in the human services*. New York: Wiley.

Risley, T. R., and Reynolds, N. J. (1970). Emphasis as a prompt for verbal imitation. *Journal of Applied Behavior Analysis, 3*, 185–190.

Welch, S. (1981). Teaching generative grammar to mentally retarded children: A review and analysis of a decade of behavioral research. *Mental Retardation, 19*, 277–284.

Whaley, D. L., and Malott, R. W. (1971). *Elementary principles of behavior*. Englewood Cliffs, NJ: Prentice-Hall.

Williams, G. C., and McReynolds, L. V. (1975). The relationship between discrimination and articulation training in children with misarticulation. *Journal of Speech and Hearing Research, 18*, 401–412.

Winokur, S. (1976). *A primer of verbal behavior: An operant view*. Englewood Cliffs, NJ: Prentice-Hall.

Chapter 7

Discrimination, Generalization, and Maintenance

In Chapter 6, the need for stimulus control procedures, including modeling, imitation, instructions, prompting, and fading, was discussed.

In Chapter 7, the following points will be described:

- The concepts of discrimination and generalization
- Discrimination training procedure
- Types of generalization
- Problems with the concept of generalization
- Response maintenance strategies

With the procedures described in the previous chapters, the clinician should be able to establish target behaviors. This does not mean, however, that the client is ready to be dismissed. Some additional procedures must be implemented for at least two reasons. The first is that when certain behaviors are trained, they may be generalized inappropriately. The second is that desirable and appropriate generalization of trained behaviors may not take place, or if it does, the responses may not be maintained. The client is ready to be dismissed only when the target behaviors are produced appropriately and maintained in the home, school, playground, workplace, supermarket, and other such natural settings.

In this chapter, the issue of how to prevent inappropriate generalization by training discrimination and how to promote appropriate generalization and eventual maintenance of target behaviors will be addressed.

DISCRIMINATION

In understanding discrimination, it is useful to contrast it with generalization. The two are opposite processes. When there is discrimination, there is no generalization. When there is generalization (appropriate or not), there is no discrimination. In an advanced stage of clinical training, discrimination and generalization are important considerations. The client's response rates must show appropriate discrimination as well as generalization.

In discrimination, different responses are given to different stimuli. In generalization, on the other hand, the same response is given to different stimuli. Different stimuli may share certain common properties, which in turn may lead to generalization. Such a generalization, however, may be entirely inappropriate, and what is expected may be discrimination (different, not the same, responses). For example, a young child who is in the process of learning the basic vocabulary may call all women "Mommy." In this case, the child has inappropriately generalized the word "Mommy" to all women because of certain similarities between them. Such inappropriate generalizations illustrate a lack of discrimination. When the child is eventually able to call only his or her mother "Mommy" and other women with different and appropriate names, the child has learned discrimination. It is a lack of generalization.

Studies of language acquisition have documented many instances of failure to discriminate. A variety of vocabulary items learned initially tend to generalize inappropriately (Dale, 1976; Owens, 1984). A child may use the word "truck" to describe all vehicles, or the word "doggie" to name all four-legged animals. Any circular stimulus may be called "moon," and any colored drink "juice." Eventually, children begin to discriminate and produce labels that are specific to stimulus classes.

Discrimination is the result of a procedure called differential reinforcement, in which a response in the presence of a stimulus is reinforced and the same response in the presence of other stimuli is extinguished (not reinforced), or even punished. As a result, the response is more likely in the presence of the stimulus associated with reinforcement and less likely in the presence of all other stimuli. In the example just given, the child may be reinforced for calling the mother "Mommy" but not for calling other women by the same name. The child may also be punished by verbal statements such as "no, she is not your Mommy" when that word is used in relation to other women. Such differential reinforcement (and punishment) is responsible for the eventual discrimination between the mother and other women.

A stimulus in the presence of which a response is reinforced is called a discriminative stimulus. It is abbreviated S^D (pronounced essdee.) The response becomes more probable in the presence of its S^D, presumably because the stimulus signals reinforcement. The stimulus in the presence of which a response is not reinforced is known as S Δ (pronounced ess-delta). When a given stimulus becomes an S^D for a particular response because of differential reinforcement, other stimuli belonging to the same class as the S^D also acquire some power to evoke the response. Indeed, this is what happens when the child begins to call all other women "Mommy," even though it is inappropriate. There are many other situations where such a phenomenon is appropriate. For example, when a child has learned the word "chair," it is appropriate to use the word in relation to chairs of different size and design. As stimuli, all chairs belong to a class, and the same response may be appropriate for all members of that class.

All stimuli, however, do not belong to a single class. There are different classes of stimuli. If all chairs form a class of stimuli, all tables form another class. Generalization of a response within a class is socially acceptable, but not across classes. What is expected across different classes of stimuli is discrimination. Different names are used for different classes of events, objects, and persons. That is discriminated responding, a result of differential reinforcement. Generalization within a class of stimuli and discrimination across classes is also the basis of *concepts*. When a child uses the word "chair" for chairs of different shape, size, design, color and texture, but uses the word "table" for tables similarly varied, it is said that the child has the concepts of chair and table. The logic can be applied to more complex conceptual behaviors. In fact, generalization and discrimination are the two most important processes underlying the learning and production of verbal behaviors (language). A language has as many concepts as there are differentiated stimulus classes.

In addition to generalization and discrimination, a process known as abstraction is also involved in the formation of complex conceptual behaviors. In fact, in order for generalization to occur across members of a class of stimuli that may be different in many ways, the response should come under the control of a single property or very few properties shared by those stimuli. When it is said that a child "knows the colors," what is meant technically is that different color naming responses are controlled by their respective single (or unique) properties of the wave lengths of stimuli. When a child has learned to say "red" appropriately, then the actual stimulus events for which the term is a response may be infinitely varied in terms of shape, size, texture, use, and so on. Consider the following stimulus events that may be "red": chair, brick, dress, sky, book, lipstick, telephone, car, carpet, Jupiter, blood. Unless a single property of these varied stimulus events (wave length) comes to control the response "red," the child cannot generalize, nor can he or she discriminate "red" from other colors. In the behavioral analysis, control over a response exerted by a single or unique stimulus property is called abstraction. Abstract stimulus control will result in appropriate generalization and discrimination.

Discrimination Training in Clinical Work

After certain behaviors have been established in the clinic, there are times when discrimination training is needed. In essence, whenever there is unacceptable generalization (overgeneralization), discrimination training is needed. Clinical studies have observed overgeneralization, particularly in language training (Guess and Baer, 1973; Hegde and McConn, 1981). For example, a child who has just been trained to produce the plural /s/ correctly may overgeneralize it to nouns that take plural /z/. Any of the trained plural morphemes may also overgeneralize to singular stimulus conditions or irregular plural forms. Trained singular verbal auxiliary (is) may be produced in contexts where the plural form (are) is appropriate. When the regular past tense is trained, it might overgeneralize to the irregular past tense. In situations such as these, discrimination training is needed so that different and appropriate responses are produced in relation to different stimulus classes.

The procedure to eliminate such overgeneralization is the same that produces discrimination: differential reinforcement. A response in the presence of one stimulus is reinforced, whereas the same response in the presence of another stimulus is not reinforced. In training discrimination between singular and plural noun labels, the clinician has two sets of stimuli, singular and plural objects. When singular objects are presented, the singular label is reinforced, and while plural objects are presented, the plural form is reinforced. In this procedure, each stimulus has its S^D and $S\Delta$. The picture of a single book, for instance, is an S^D for "book" (reinforced), but it is an $S\Delta$ for "books" (not reinforced; may be even punished). A picture of two or more books, on the other hand, is an S^D for "books" but an $S\Delta$ for "book." Through such differential programming of consequences that match the stimulus conditions with expected responses, appropriately discriminated response classes can be generated. The same discrete trial procedure described in Chapter 5 can be used in discrimination training.

It must be noted that most clinical training procedures involve differential reinforcement. The procedure of reinforcing correct responses and extinguishing or punishing incorrect responses is essentially the same as differential reinforcement technique.

GENERALIZATION

Generalization is the term currently used by many researchers and clinicians to describe the final goal of treatment programs. It is said that behaviors trained in clinical settings should generalize to natural environments. However, the term generalization poses some significant problems in the context of applied research and treatment. Therefore, it is more appropriate to consider response maintenance as the final target of clinical intervention strategies. However, when generalization does take place, it can serve a useful clinical purpose. Different types of generalization will be considered first, and then a number of maintenance strategies will be described.

Generalization has a stimulus dimension and a response dimension. It is the basis upon which some new learning is demonstrated without additional conditioning. Generalization refers to either an extension of learning to new situations and stimuli, or new responses based upon old learning. There are different types of generalization, which will be briefly described.

Stimulus Generalization

Stimulus generalization is evident when a response learned in relation to one stimulus is evoked by stimuli that were not involved in the original conditioning situation. Most of the basic research information on stimulus generalization can be summarized as follows.

1. All learning necessarily takes place in a certain situational context, which is nothing but a bundle of stimuli. It may be recalled that stimulus variables are a part of the contingency, and stimuli acquire the power to evoke responses because of reinforcement contingencies.
2. No stimulus is a discrete entity. All stimuli are generic, in the sense that they are members of larger classes. A large number of stimuli may fall into a class because they share certain properties such as size, color, shape, or texture. Stimuli may also form classes on the basis of use, which means that people act upon them in similar manners. Different items of furniture, for example, may fall into a class on this basis.
3. Initial learning necessarily takes place in relation to one or a few stimuli. The clinician teaching the word "ball" to a child uses a specific ball or a few pictures of balls. When the client later comes in contact with other (novel) balls, the response may be likely. The

greater the similarity between the training and the novel stimuli, higher the chances of stimulus generalization.

4. As the difference between the training and the novel stimuli increases, the response rate decreases. In the example just given, if the clinician were to present progressively different balls to the client, the response "ball" would eventually diminish because of an increasing (and eventually extreme) difference between the training stimulus and the new stimulus. This phenomenon is known as the generalization gradient. In laboratory research, generalization is measured in the absence of reinforcement during the presentation of stimuli that are progressively different from the training stimulus. In this sense, measures of generalization are similar to measures of extinction.

5. Although people (and animals) show stimulus generalization, it is not an activity of the subject. Clients do not generalize, but untrained stimuli evoke responses from them. However, it is dependent upon a number of manipulable variables, such as stimulus variety, and reinforcement schedule.

6. Although the clinician programs initial learning in relation to specific stimuli, the actual learning takes place in a larger stimulus context, which includes the entire physical setting, the therapy room, the verbal antecedents of responses and the clinician. All these factors lead to different types of stimulus generalization.

TYPES OF STIMULUS GENERALIZATION

Physical Stimulus Generalization. Although responses are typically controlled by a bundle of discriminative stimuli, there are standard stimuli for most responses. For example, the verbal response "ball" may have a variety of actual balls, pictures of balls, or the printed word "ball" as its standard physical stimuli. In clinical training, certain pictures or actual balls may be used. Should there be any generalization, the word "ball" may be evoked by pictures of balls or actual balls that were not used in training. This phenomenon is described as the physical-stimulus generalization in this book. It can also be called standard-stimulus generalization.

The physical stimulus generalization is evident when a learned response is evoked by standard stimuli that were not a part of the original learning condition. If a client were to generalize the target behaviors to most of the standard stimuli, training time and effort could be minimized.

Verbal Stimulus Generalization. In the treatment of communicative disorders, verbal stimuli provided by the clinician play a major role. In most language treatment programs, the clinician asks questions such as "what is this?" and "what do you see?" or makes requests such as "tell me about this" and "say what I say." As a function of training, these questions, requests, and other verbal devices can come to evoke the target responses from the client. Such verbal devices are antecedents in the sense that they become a part of the S^Ds evoking target behaviors.

Normally, the same verbal behaviors have multiple antecedents. A target behavior such as "the boy is running" may be evoked by "what is the boy doing?" or "what is happening in the picture?" or "tell me about the boy," and so on. In training, a particular antecedent may be used consistently. Verbal stimulus generalization is evident when target behaviors are evoked by verbal antecedents that were not used in training.

Verbal antecedent generalization is very important for clinical speech-language training. Speech itself is probably the most pervasive stimulus for speech. Unless natural speech stimuli become SDs for clinically trained speech, the success of the training progam remains questionable. When a child sees a ball, or wants a ball, or has something to say about a ball in the natural environment, he or she should not need the same triggering stimuli that were used in clinical training.

Physical Setting Generalization. All treatment necessarily takes place in a certain physical setting. Mostly, treatment is done in small and isolated rooms with minimum furnishings and equipment that are arranged in a relatively constant fashion. Most therapeutic settings are unlike the client's natural environment, and as such, they are discriminated. Discriminated therapeutic settings are desirable and sometimes even necessary for initial learning because they are devoid of competing stimuli. However, when responses are reinforced in discriminated settings, they become "attached" to those settings. Target behaviors produced reliably in treatment settings may not be produced in natural environments.

When responses trained in one physical setting are produced in nontreatment settings, physical setting generalization has occurred. For example, after having taught the correct production of /r/ in the context of ten single words, the clinician might take the client to another room, outdoors, or the client's home. In these settings, the clinician might try to evoke the same ten words with the help of the very same pictures used during training. If the client uses the target phoneme, physical setting generalization will have been demonstrated.

Audience Generalization. One of the most powerful discriminative stimuli for speech is the presence of other people. In behavioral analysis, people are called audience when they serve as discriminative stimuli for speech (Winokur, 1976). Speech is reinforced by other people, and by virtue of this fact, people themselves acquire discriminative stimulus value. This phenomenon gives rise to what can be described as audience generalization.

Audience generalization can be described as a phenomenon in which responses trained or typically evoked by a given audience are evoked by other audiences not involved in training. The clinician who reinforces a target behavior quickly becomes the audience for that behavior. Family members and other people, not having reinforced the behavior, may not serve the role of audience. When they do, audience generalization is evident.

Factorial Stimulus Generalization. The four types of stimulus generalization (physical stimulus, verbal stimulus, physical setting, and audience) may not always be independent of each other. In most cases, different types of stimulus generalizations are concurrently active. They can be separately manipulated, however. When a trained behavior does not show stimulus generalization, the specific type of stimulus generalization that has failed must be investigated.

When the correct production of a grammatic feature, a plural morpheme for example, generalizes to the home situation, a more complex form of generalization, called factorial generalization, may have occurred. It is very likely that the client is responding to plural objects that are different from any encountered in the treatment sessions. In all probability, the child is responding to family members and not the clinician. It is also possible that verbal antecedents of those target responses are different. Therefore, the client's correct production of the plural morpheme at home is a product of all types of stimulus generalization. The responses may be the same ("books" and "cups," for example), but they are emitted in a new setting and, in relation to stimuli not used in treatment, are evoked by people other than the clinician, and are triggered by verbal stimuli that were not a part of treatment. In essence, it is a combination of standard physical stimulus, physical setting, verbal stimulus, and audience generalization. In this book, this type of generalization is called factorial stimulus generalization.

Factorial stimulus generalization is evident when a response learned with one set of antecedents in a given physical setting is evoked by new and multiple antecedents in new settings. The term factorial simply suggests that different stimulus factors are simultaneously varied. This type of generalization is probably common in everyday situations. It is very desirable from the clinical standpoint.

Response Generalization

Stimulus generalization deals with untrained or novel stimuli, but the same (trained) response form. Response generalization, on the other hand, deals with new (untrained) responses.

When a response has been learned, it can serve as a basis for new responses. A child who has been taught to cooperate with other children in play situations may also learn to smile more. A child who receives language training and thus becomes verbally more proficient may also show increased social activity. A man who has his very high vocal pitch treated successfully may speak more in conversational situations. A young stuttering womam who becomes relatively fluent as a result of therapy may begin to seek the company of young men. Each of these examples has a response trained by the clinician, and a new response based upon that "old" learning. This phenomenon is known as response generalization.

Typically, response generalization has been defined as the production of new and therefore unreinforced responses similar to those that have been reinforced. It is generally assumed that the new responses are evoked by the same stimuli that were involved in the original learning. It is often said that in stimulus generalization, new stimuli evoke the old response, whereas in response generalization, the old stimuli evoke new responses. When this is the case, stimuli change in stimulus generalization and responses change in response generalization.

The standard operant descriptions of response generalization pose some significant problems when applied to verbal behaviors. The majority of clinical studies in which verbal response generalization has been documented involved changes in both stimulus and response variables. Take, for instance, the earlier example of a client trained to produce the plural morpheme in words such as "cups" and "books." In order to assess generalization of this target behavior, the clinician might present a variety of untrained stimulus items such as "hats" and "plates." A correct production of "hats" and "plates" would mean there was some generalization. But what kind of generalization is this?

To take another example from treatment of articulation disorders, suppose a child has been trained in the correct production of /f/ in the context of a certain number of single words. The clinician then might try to evoke some untrained words in order to assess generalization. If the child were to produce such untrained words as "fire," "fish," and "foot," the child will have demonstrated generalization. But again, what kind of generalization?

It is obvious that when the untrained pictures or words were presented, stimuli changed. But one feature of the stimulus complex (which is supposed to evoke the target response) was common to the trained and untrained stimuli in both instances. The response also changed, for the particular words containing the plural morpheme or the target phoneme were not involved in training. Nevertheless, the generalized response was not entirely new: It contained either the trained plural /s/ or the target phoneme (f). This means that it was not a pure form of either stimulus or response generalization, but was actually both. For this reason, the term intraverbal generalization is suggested here to describe the kinds of posttreatment changes that may take place in verbal behaviors.

Intraverbal Generalization

Posttreatment changes in verbal behaviors include either a substitution of old responses by new responses of the same class, or an expansion of the entire response topography. The term intraverbal generalization refers to generalized verbal response substitutions and topographic expansions.

A client who has been trained on such sentences as "the boy is running" and "the boy is walking" may generalize the target *is* not only to sentences such as "the boy is eating" but also to sentences such as "the girl is writing," "the man is washing," and "the rabbit is hopping." Each of the generalized responses illustrates the substitution process: New nouns and verbs were substituted for trained nouns and verbs. This type of generalization contains some constant responses, one or more substituted responses, many new stimulus elements, and one constant property of the stimulus complex. The stimulus property that is constant is discriminative of the auxiliary *is*. The property discriminative of the definite article is also constant, but that is beside the point.

The process of generalized expansion of trained verbal responses can be illustrated as follows. Suppose the client who has learned to use the plural /s/ in the context of single words produces untrained responses such as "I see two books," "books are here," "look at the cups," and "where are the cups?" These are generalized verbal expansions. Similarly, if the phoneme /f/ trained only in the context of single words generalizes to appropriate phrases and sentences, another instance has occurred of generalized expansion of response topography. It is important to note that intraverbal generalization necessarily includes new discriminative stimulus control.

Many langauge training studies have demonstrated that it is possible to induce intraverbal generalization. It is known that clients are typically able to use trained grammatical features in the context of untrained responses. This might result in either substituted or expanded verbal responses.

Intraverbal generalization, like stimulus generalization, can help minimize training time and effort. When it does occur, it may be one of the best forms of generalization, since it includes new and expanded responses as well as additional discriminative stimulus control.

Response Mode Generalization

In speech and language training, targeted response mode may be verbal or nonverbal. The client may be asked either to produce speech or language behaviors or to nonverbally respond to verbal stimuli. For example, a client in articulation training may be asked either to produce the target phoneme in words, or to distinguish the target phoneme from the nontarget phoneme when it is produced by the clinician. In the latter procedure, the client may raise the right hand when the target sound is heard ("radio") and the left hand when the nontarget sound is heard ("wadio").

In language training, the client may be trained either to say certain utterances, or respond nonverbally when verbal signals are given. For example, a child may be trained to produce the possessive morphemes in words such as "Mommy's hat" and "Daddy's coat" or to differentially point to appropriate pictures. There are more complex examples. A client may be trained to either say sentences such as "please open the door" or to actually open the door when that request is made.

The frequently asked question in this context is whether one mode of responding generalizes to the other. For example, when a child is able to differentially (and nonverbally) signal the productions of a target and a nontarget phoneme, will the child be able to produce the target phoneme? When a client is able to correctly point to pictures of "Mommy's hat" and "Daddy's coat," will he or she be able to produce those responses? Some clinicians believe that nonverbal responding to verbal stimuli must be trained before training the production of those verbal responses. Others believe that nonverbal response training may not be needed, and when accomplished, may not automatically result in productive speech.

The question of response mode generalization is still a controversial issue. In the field of communicative disorders, it is not clear whether it is a reliable phenomenon. Therefore, the response mode generalization can be tentatively defined as the possibility that a response trained in one mode would be produced in another mode. The two most commonly described modes are verbal and nonverbal.

When nonverbal communicative behaviors are targeted, it is the common practice to describe them as "comprehension." The client is said to comprehend the difference between /r/ and /w/ or that between the singular and the plural forms of words. But "comprehension" refers to a mental state inaccessible to observation or measurement. When a client responds appropriately when asked to "show cups" or "open the door," the clinician infers a mental state of "comprehension." It is obviously inferred from the appropriate nonverbal responses of pointing to cups and opening the door.

The issue, then, is whether trained response modes generalize to untrained modes. Investigators have tried to assess generalization either of trained nonverbal responses to verbal productions, or of trained verbal productions to nonverbal responses. Most of the studies have been done in the areas of language and articulation disorders (Connell and McReynolds, 1981; Guess and Baer, 1973; Keller and Bucher, 1979; Williams and McReynolds, 1976). A majority of studies have shown that nonverbal response training may not result in the production of verbal responses, whereas verbal response training may produce both verbal and corresponding nonverbal responses.

The available evidence concerning response mode generalization suggests that it is better to first train production of communicative behaviors. Whenever necessary, nonverbal responding to verbal stimuli can be probed. If the client is not able to respond nonverbally to targeted verbal stimuli, then those responses may be trained.

CONCURRENT STIMULUS-RESPONSE GENERALIZATION

The final form of generalization to be described is probably the most complex, and it includes all forms of generalization discussed so far. Factorial stimulus generalization, which is a combination of multiple types of stimulus generalization, was discussed earlier. When factorial stimulus generalization is combined with response generalization, concurrent stimulus-response generalization is present.

Concurrent stimulus-response generalization is evident when both the stimulus and response variables change subsequent to original learning. The change may be sudden, simultaneous, or achieved over a period of time, but the result is a complex form of stimulus and response generalization in which a variety of new stimuli control forms of responses that were never trained.

Concurrent stimulus response generalizations can be illustrated from a clinical standpoint. Suppose a clinician teaches a child to produce the possessive /s/ in the context of short phrases ("cat's tail," "Pat's coat," and so on). The child then goes home and begins to produce such untrained sentences as "here is cat's food," "rabbit's ears," and "I see the parrot's cage." Assume that these verbal responses on the part of the child were preceded by various questions and comments from the mother. In this case, the child will have shown a complex combination of stimulus and response generalization of the possessive morpheme.

The responses produced at home may show concurrent stimulus-response generalization of the following kinds: (1) setting generalization, because they were produced in a nontraining situation; (2) verbal-stimulus generalization, because the verbal antecedents may not have been a part of training; (3) standard physical-stimulus generalization, because the stimuli that triggered the responses may not have been involved in training; (4) audience generalization, because the mother was a new audience for those responses; and (5) response generalization of the intraverbal variety, because of additions to, and expansions of, the response topography.

If the concurrent stimulus-response generalization occurs, it is most beneficial from the clinical standpoint. Clinically trained responses must be produced in various nontreatment settings, triggered by natural physical stimuli, in response to everyday verbal antecedents, in the presence of people the client comes in contact with, and in expanded and novel forms.

PROBLEMS WITH THE CONCEPT OF GENERALIZATION

As a laboratory phenomenon, generalization has no major problems, since it simply summarizes some observations: that a controlling relationship between new stimuli and old responses or old stimuli and new responses may be evident following conditioning. Problems are encountered only when this phenomenon is set up as the ultimate goal of clinical interventions. The essence of the argument to be presented in this section is that the phenomenon of generalization has been conceptually and methodologically distorted in the context of clinical intervention. When generalization does occur, it can serve as a basis for further clinical programming, but it cannot be the final, programmed goal.

In the laboratory, generalization is a measure of a declining rate of response under conditions of changing stimuli and absence of reinforcement. Eventually, the response will be extinguished. In a sense, generalization may be an early stage of extinction. How long the response rate will continue in the absence of reinforcement will depend upon a number of factors, including the nature of the novel stimuli presented, the schedule, the amount and the quality of reinforcement, and the length and amount of training. As a function of these variables, generalized responding may be high or low, and may continue for relatively long or short durations, but in the end there is extinction.

One of the basic tenets of behaviorism is that all responses are maintained by their consequences. Generalization, however, is a short-term phenomenon of response rate in the absence of consequences. It lasts as long as it does only because of the discriminative stimulus value. However, the discriminative stimulus value can control responses only temporarily, because it is a progressively decreasing phenomenon. As novel stimuli that are more and more different from the training stimuli are encountered, the discriminative value of those stimuli decreases. Consequently, the response faces extinction unless reinforcement contingencies come to play to reestablish and broaden the discriminative stimulus control, and thus take over the response rate.

In clinical settings, generalization has been considered the final goal because it has seemed to be what is needed. The clinician cannot go on reinforcing the target behaviors because he or she will not be there in the client's natural environment. It has been thought that the solution is generalization, because generalized responses (as long as they last) do not require reinforcement. In clinical contexts, this amounts to a presumption that response rates will be maintained indefinitely in the absence of reinforcement contingencies. Obviously, this is impossible from the standpoint of behaviorism. Therefore, the phenomenon of generalization, as observed in the laboratory, cannot be the ultimate goal of clinical intervention programs. Whenever it is treated as such, two major problems have emerged.

First, this highly desirable final goal of clinical treatment has been elusive. Clinical studies have observed some stimulus and response generalization, but often the extent is negligible. Some trained behaviors are produced some of the time in certain naturalistic situations. More typically, however, behaviors that are produced reliably in the clinic are not generalized to nonclinical settings.

Second, and more important, generalized responses may not last in the natural environment. That is, even when responses do generalize, they may not be maintained over time. This is not surprising, since generalization is not an indefinite process. Generalized but not maintained responses show that generalization can only lead to extinction.

The Typical Strategy

Having encountered those two major problems in applied settings, clinical researchers have suggested that it is necessary to program generalization. Since generalization may not automatically follow training, and when it does it may be only temporary, additional steps must be taken to make it happen reliably and last indefinitely. In their review of studies involving generalization in behavioral research, Stokes and Baer (1977) have found a number of tactics used to measure, promote, or program generalization. The strategies identified by them include train and hope, sequential modification, natural maintaining contingencies, sufficient exemplars, loose training, indiscriminable contingencies, common stimuli, mediated generalization, and train "to generalize." According to Stokes and Baer (1977) train and hope and sequential modification are not programming tactics. The rest of them seek to actively program generalization.

In addition to Stokes and Baer (1977) whose review article has been very influential in recent years, many researchers have drawn clinicians' attention to the basic problem associated with generalization (Costello, 1983; Drabman, Hammer, and Rosenbaum, 1979; Ingham, 1984; Kazdin, 1984; Marholin, Siegel, and Phillips, 1976; Scott, Himadi, and Keane, 1983, among others). As a result, clinicians now are more concerned about the course of the target behaviors after the treatment program has been terminated.

A significant problem with strategies of generalization programming is that some of the assumptions underlying such an attempt may not be valid. It is possible that generalization should not be the terminal goal of clinical intervention because the term describes a decreasing rate of response, which may result in extinction. The following four assumptions are questionable as they underlie the concept of programmed generalization.

First, the very idea of programming generalization is conceptually confusing. When generalization is programmed, a temporary and declining rate of response without reinforcement is being programmed. Since the goal of treatment programs is to have a lasting rate of responses, generalization would have to be redefined as a lasting rate of response in the absence of reinforcement contingencies. It is hard to find either an empirical basis or a compelling reason for such a redefinition.

Second, programming generalization means that lasting response rates in the absence of reinforcement contingencies are expected. Such an expectation would violate one of the most important principles of behaviorism (Ferster, Culbertson, and Boren, 1975; Kalish, 1981; Skinner, 1953, 1969, 1974). Any behavior lasts only because of the lasting contingencies. If behaviors are to be maintained, contingencies must also be maintained, and therefore, generalization (as a decreasing response rate in the absence of contingencies) should not be the goal of clinical intervention.

Third, some tactics of generalization offer a de facto definition of that phenomenon in terms of a response rate reinforced in other situations or by other persons. One of the tactics of generalization, for example, is to have the response come under natural reinforcement contingencies. Another strategy is to treat generalized response as the target and reinforce its occurrence. Such strategies confuse generalization with treatment done outside the clinical settings. It is not clear why reinforcement of responses in clinical settings should be considered treatment, whereas the same thing done outside the clinic is considered generalization.

Fourth, the concept of programmed generalization seems to be based upon the questionable assumption that the only contingencies of importance are the ones administered by the clinician. When the clinician withdraws the contingencies, the response is supposedly maintained because of generalization. Behaviorism asserts that response maintenance is also due to operant conditioning (Skinner, 1953). It means that responses are maintained only when reinforced. Whether the reinforcing agent is the clinician or some other person(s) is irrelevant.

The foregoing reasons suggest that to conceptualize the final target of clinical treatment in terms of generalization is inconsistent with behaviorism. As Drabman and colleagues have pointed out, "the current practice of subjective reference to a variety of phenomena as generalization is unacceptable" (1979, p. 204). Scott and colleagues (1983) have also stated that many techniques intended to extend the treatment effects to nontreatment conditions are "not always consistent with the process of generalization. Using a single experimental term to describe a number of different clinical phenomena can only invite confusion and imprecision" (p. 118). There is no compelling reason why the term generalization should not be restored to its original meaning in the applied context.

Generalization Versus Response Maintenance

The final target of clinical intervention is not generalization, but response maintenance in natural environments. After the treatment contingencies are terminated, responses must be maintained by contingencies operative in the client's everyday situations. If natural contingencies are defective, and often they may be, then steps must be taken to make sure that they are effective. Within this conceptual framework, there will be no attempt to have the target behaviors produced in the absence of reinforcement contingencies (generalization). Instead, the clinician will focus upon the problems involved in contingency management in nonclinical settings.

When the transition from the clinic to natural environments is being made, generalization can help, however. There are some programming techniques that are consistent with the true nature of generalization. When generalization does take place, it can serve as a basis for maintenance strategies that help strengthen the responses in natural environments. Obviously, those strategies must be instituted before generalized responses are extinguished.

MAINTENANCE STRATEGIES

Responses are not maintained after the termination of treatment, possibly because of two reasons. First, factors relating to treatment may be discriminated, which means that target behaviors are likely to be exhibited only in the treatment setting. Second, the natural environmental might still contain S^Ds for undesirable behaviors and no S^Ds for desirable ones. The undesirable behaviors may receive reinforcement while the desirable behaviors are extinguished. The clinician's task in promoting response maintenance is to reverse the process: The natural environment should become discriminative of the target behaviors and should not support the undesirable behaviors.

Contingency management for the sake of response maintenance involves manipulation of all three aspects of that contingency: stimuli, responses, and consequences. In this sense, it is not unlike treatment offered by the clinician. The single most important difference between treatment and maintenance is the locus of response control. During treatment, responses are controlled in the treatment setting by the clinician. During maintenance, the same responses are controlled by people in a client's everyday situations. Thus, a shift in the locus of response control is the heart of maintenance strategies.

It might appear logical to think of response maintenance strategies after the behaviors have been clinically established. However, several factors suggest that response maintenance must be planned from the very beginning. There are a number of stimulus, response, and contingency related issues that deserve consideration before, during, and after treatment. Maintenance strategy will be described in terms of (1) stimulus manipulations, (2) response considerations, and (3) consequence manipulations.

Stimulus Manipulations

The kinds of stimuli used in training target responses can have an effect on the initial generalization and subsequent maintenance of those responses. Neutral stimuli used in training eventually become discriminative stimuli capable of evoking target responses. Therefore, stimulus considerations are important in planning for generalization and maintenance. The logic underlying stimulus manipulations is that what is needed is a transition from clinical stimulus control to extra-clinical stimulus control of target behaviors. Thus, shifting the stimulus control is the central theme of stimulus manipulation strategies. The following suggestions can be useful in this regard.

SELECT STANDARD STIMULI
FROM NATURAL ENVIRONMENTS

Typically, stimuli for target behaviors are selected somewhat arbitrarily. Most stimulus materials used in training happen to be present in the clinic. Often, commercially prepared stimulus materials may be used. These materials may or may not be particularly relevant to the individual client being trained. Response maintenance may be enhanced when stimuli used in training are present in the client's environment. When stimuli selected from natural environment are used in training, they acquire discriminative stimulus value. Later, when the client faces those stimuli at home, the production of target behaviors is more likely.

Clinicians often use pictures in training speech and language behaviors. Even a cursory glance at commercially available stimulus pictures suggest that their quality and the extent to which they represent true objects vary tremendously. Pictures selected from popular magazines may be more representative of the real objects than some of the commercially available materials. It is more helpful to use real objects themselves if that is possible. There is some evidence that in language training, real objects promote better generalization to home situations than do pictures (Faw, Reid, Schepis, Fitzgerald, and Welty, 1981; Welch and Pear, 1980). Another advantage of real objects is that they can be used to represent events because they are more manipulable than pictures. In teaching *verb+ing*, for example, toy trucks, cars, and several other objects can be used to demonstrate movement. Whether selected stimuli are pictures or objects, they should be a part of the client's environment.

Careful selection of stimulus materials that are present in the client's environment is probably more crucial in treating articulation and language disorders than in treating voice or fluency disorders. The ideal strategy may be to ask the parents to bring in selected stimulus materials from home. The child may bring his or her own toys and other belongings to the therapy situation, which may then serve as stimuli for the target behaviors under training. When this is done, the discriminative stimuli used in training are carried back to the home situation.

SELECT COMMON VERBAL ANTECEDENTS

In addition to real objects and events as stimuli, communicative behaviors also have their unique verbal antecedents. In many cases, verbal antecedents may be the sole triggering stimuli of language behaviors. Questions, requests, comments, suggestions, hints, prompts, modeling, and so on are potentially effective verbal antecedents of target behaviors.

Some verbal antecedents may be more frequently encountered in everyday situations than some of the antecedents used in clinical situations. For example, modeling, leading to imitative responses, is not as frequently associated with verbal responses as are questions and requests. Therefore, when modeling is used, the clinician must fade it out as soon as possible and use the kinds of antecedents that may be found more frequently in natural settings. Questions and requests such as "what is happening?" "what is the girl doing?" and "tell me about this" are more natural than hints and prompts, which are provided in everyday situations only when reponses fail in the first instance.

VARY AUDIENCE-ANTECEDENT CONTROLS

Because it is the clinician who initially reinforces correct responses, he or she will quickly become the discriminative audience for those responses. As a result, responses are more likely to be correct in the presence of the clinician, and less likely in the presence of other people, including family members. The clinician is not the typical audience of verbal responses, and therefore, family members and other persons should eventually be involved in the training sessions so that they can also become the discriminative audience. Parents and siblings can take part in training sessions. Initially, they may just observe the clinician and the training procedure being implemented. Soon, they may be asked to administer some stimulus items. Eventually, they may be trained to reinforce correct responses, in which case the other persons can also be expected to acquire discriminative stimulus value. The correct responses may then be more likely in their presence.

Student observers, other student clinicians, or colleagues of the clinician can serve as audience. These persons can also take part in the training sequence the way family members can. When this is done systematically, the exclusive control exerted by a clinician on target behaviors is reduced and a broader control is instituted.

There is some evidence that a certain amount of initial generalization to persons not involved in training can take place (Faw et al., 1981; Hegde, 1980; Hegde et al., 1979). There is no assurance however, that generalized responses are always maintained. Generalized responses may be maintained only when natural reinforcing contingencies gain control over them.

VARY PHYSICAL SETTING CONTROLS

The physical setting in which training takes place can also quickly acquire discriminative stimulus value. But in more natural settings such as home, school, or office, the target behaviors may be absent. To overcome this problem, the clinician should vary the physical setting of treatment so that multiple settings come to control target responses.

A desirable strategy is to hold training sessions in different rooms that vary in size and setup. As target behaviors become more and more stable, training can be less formal, and as a result, progressively less formal situations may be appropriate for contingency management. Contingency management in more naturalistic settings will have to be subtle, however. This point will be discussed again in a later section.

A few studies have shown that when training takes place in multiple settings, or in more naturalistic settings, there is usually better generalization of target behaviors (Carr and Kologinsky, 1983; Handleman, 1979; Hegde and McConn, 1981; McGee, Krantz, Mason, and McClannahan, 1983). When different physical settings are used, an important aspect of stimulus control of resposes will have been broadened.

In some clinical populations, such as autistic children, the physical setting and other stimulus conditions used in training seem to exert unusually circumscribed control on target behaviors (Lovaas, Koegel, Simmons, and Stevens-Long, 1973; Rincover and Koegel, 1975). Stutterers also tend to exhibit tight stimulus control of fluent and dysfluent behaviors. Compared with nonclinical populations, it is possible that clinical populations that need explicit management of reinforcement contingencies in order to learn any kind of behavior are likely to come under relatively strict stimulus controls. Thus, varying physical setting controls is an important aspect of stimulus manipulations designed to promote generalization and maintenance.

Response Considerations

A number of generalization and maintenance strategies relate to certain characteristics of target responses. Some responses may have a better chance of being reinforced and thus maintained in natural environments than some others a clinician might arbitrarily select for training. This suggests that maintenance considerations are important even at the stage of target behavior selection. In this sense, maintenance is not something to be considered only after target behaviors are established.

SELECT CLIENT-SPECIFIC RESPONSES

Target responses are often selected because developmental norms suggest them, or because most clients seem to need them in order to be able to interact socially. However, such responses may or may not have special relevance to given clients. It may be more meaningful to select target responses that are specific to the individual client's needs as assessed by an examination of that client's particular environment. Nonverbal children may be taught labels of colors or furniture items, but such responses may not have a pragmatic relevance. Instead, such children can be taught labels of toys, food items, or clothing articles. There is some evidence that such responses generalize more readily than labels of furniture items or body parts (Duker and Morsink, 1984). Such responses help the client gain better control over the environment. Once generalized, those responses are likely to be reinforced at home and other natural settings.

This approach of selecting client-specific target behaviors was described in Chapter 3. Consult that chapter for additional information.

SELECT MULTIPLE EXEMPLARS

A target behavior is a collection of multiple responses, all being controlled by the same or similar contingency. Each response is an example of a given response class. In order for target responses to be produced and reinforced in everyday situations, an adequate number of responses from the class targeted for training must be sampled.

The number of responses needed to obtain generalization, maintenance, or both varies with clients and types of behaviors under training. Most often, the number of exemplars needed in a given situation is determined empirically. That is, a clinician teaches a few exemplars and probes for generalization, which can serve as a basis for maintenance strategies. If there is no generalization, then additional numbers of exemplars are taught (Guess and Baer, 1973; Hegde, 1980; Hegde and Gierut, 1979; Hegde et al., 1979; Stokes and Baer, 1977). Traditionally, generalization of some sort has been the basis for judging the necessary number of exemplars to be taught in a given case. Several studies have shown that some language behaviors can generalize only after a few exemplars are trained (Stokes and Baer, 1977; Hegde et al., 1979). When sufficient numbers of exemplars are trained, the resulting generalization can provide a basis for a contingency-based maintenance strategy.

REINFORCE COMPLEX RESPONSE TOPOGRAPHIES

In many cases, responses are initially trained at simple topographical levels such as single words or short phrases. Responses may not be produced or maintained in everyday situations simply because naturally occurring topographies were not reinforced by the clinician. Both in the clinic and at home, target behaviors produced during conversational speech must be reinforced.

In some cases, clinicians simply continue to train target behaviors at simpler, more manageable topographical levels. Training may not proceed to more complex levels. Monitoring and reinforcing speech and language target responses in conversational speech is difficult and needs sharp observational skills. This difficult task must be accomplished if responses are to be generalized and maintained.

When responses are trained at more complex topographic levels, the intraverbal generalization may occur more readily. Since, by definition, intraverbal generalization involves connected speech, target responses must be trained at this level of response topography to achieve it.

Contingency Manipulations

Contingency manipulation is involved in all kinds of maintenance strategies. Although contingency management in natural environments is the most critical factor, there are some techniques that when used during training sessions can also promote generalization and maintenance.

USE INTERMITTENT REINFORCEMENT SCHEDULES

A number of clinical studies have shown that intermittent reinforcement schedules help generate target responses that may be maintained over longer periods of time than those that are reinforced continuously (Kazdin, 1984; Kazdin and Polster, 1973; Stokes and Baer, 1977). When target behaviors have increased above the baseline to a considerable extent, the schedule of reinforcement may be shifted from a continuous to an intermittent one. Initially, an intermittent schedule that permits a relatively high level of reinforcement (such as an FR2) may be appropriate. In gradual steps, the schedule may be stretched so that progressively greater number of responses go unreinforced.

Whenever possible, variable ratio schedules must be used during the latter stages of training. In everyday situations, reinforcers are more likely to come on a variable ratio. Sometimes, a few responses are reinforced; at other times many responses may go unreinforced. Variable ratios might help minimize discrimination between treatment and nontreatment conditions.

During the final phases of treatment, the client must be able to tolerate a fairly large response reinforcement ratio. Occasional reinforcers should be sufficient to maintain target responses.

USE CONDITIONED REINFORCERS

As discussed in Chapter 4, it is sometimes necessary to use primary reinforcers (food and other consumables) in case of clients who have not had a productive verbal history. It was also pointed out that a primary reinforcer may not support generalization or maintenance. Since most classes of verbal behaviors are reinforced by social reinforcers, it is most appropriate to use attention, approval, and praise to strengthen communicative responses.

Even when primary reinforcers are necessary, conditioned reinforcers must always be used so that eventually the former can be faded out while responses on the latter are maintained. Whenever possible, one of the best strategies is to use conditioned generalized reinforcers (tokens) that are backed up by a variety of reinforcers.

DELAY REINFORCEMENT

In clinical situations, the importance of immediately reinforcing target responses is usually emphasized. On the other hand, in everyday situations, reinforcers are often delayed. This can also encourage discrimination between clinical and everyday situations. Therefore, it has been suggested that delayed reinforcement may be one of the maintenance strategies (Kazdin, 1984; Stokes and Baer, 1977).

Delayed reinforcement is not an efficient method to use during the early stages of training when target responses are being shaped or increased from a very low operant level. Immediate reinforcement is necessary at this stage of treatment. Once the response has been well established, however, the delivery of reinforcers may be delayed. When this technique is used, the durations of delay must be increased gradually.

TRAIN "SIGNIFICANT OTHERS" IN CONTINGENCY MANAGEMENT

Perhaps the most important factor in maintenance is the presence or absence of appropriate consequences for behaviors in the client's natural environment. In accordance with the basic principles of behaviorism, the best way of ensuring response maintenance is to make sure that the client behaviors are indeed reinforced in natural environments.

The critical aspect of this strategy of maintenance is to shift the loci of response control. If target responses are controlled only in the clinic, they are likely to be emitted only in that setting. If the everyday environment is also a controlling environment, then those responses may be produced there. Therefore, the clinician must train the "significant others" in clients' lives. The training must be focused upon contingency management. The persons to be trained might be parents, caretakers, spouses, siblings, teachers, friends, colleagues, relatives, and others who come in contact with the client on a regular basis. With child clients, parents, siblings, babysitters, and grandparents may be the primary people to be trained. With school age children, it is often useful to train the classroom teacher and close friends. With adult clients, spouses, friends, and some colleagues may be the primary people. Training caretakers and other staff is important with institutionalized clients.

Who should be trained in contingency management is decided on an individual basis. The people the client spends the most time with are the primary target for training. The kinds of interactions the client engages in are also an important consideration. Those with whom the client spends much time interacting verbally are obviously more significant than those with whom the interactions are typically nonverbal.

Initially, the clinician can ask the family members to sit in on the treatment sessions. It is helpful to have people observe a few sessions before they are trained. The target responses are clearly identified for the observers, so that they know what is taught and what they should expect at home. They should be told of stimulus conditions and how to vary them, and must be encouraged to take careful note of contingencies and how they are managed. After a few sessions of observation, the clinician might then ask them to administer some of the treatment trials in the clinic under his or her supervision. The clinician must make sure other persons are able to administer contingencies response contingently.

A number of investigators have directly trained parents and peers to serve as therapists for children exhibiting a variety of problem behaviors (Colletti and Harris, 1977; Graziano, 1978; Koegel, Glahn, and Nieminen, 1978; O'Dell, 1974; Schumaker and Sherman, 1978). Similar procedures can be used in training peers, family members, and other persons to maintain behaviors trained by clinicians.

Family members and others should begin to manage the contingencies in their everyday situations as soon as possible. They should reinforce desirable target behaviors while withholding reinforcers for undesirable behaviors. If necessary, appropriate punishing contingencies should be programmed for undesirable behaviors. It is possible that in some cases, appropriate communicative behaviors taught in the clinic are not maintained in natural environments because in those environments the incompatible, undesirable behaviors are still being reinforced. For example, if a nonverbal child continues to receive reinforcement for gestures at home, the verbal responses trained in the clinic may not be produced at home. When it is clear that the child has an alternative verbal response, the incompatible nonverbal response should not be reinforced at home and other situations.

In order for the home management of contingencies to be effective, the clinician will have to determine whether other persons are indeed managing the contingencies. This poses significant methodologic problems. The clinician may have to ask the parents and others to tape record some of the verbal interactions to determine whether the contingencies are dispensed as expected. Sometimes, the clinician may have to visit those natural settings to see if the target behaviors are being reinforced. A limitation of these strategies is that other persons may act as expected while taping, or when the clinician is present, but not at other times. However, this may not be a serious limitation after all, because when parents are asked to tape verbal interactions frequently enough, the chances of home management of contingencies may increase just because of this requirement.

REINFORCE GENERALIZED RESPONSES

Traditionally, generalized responses are not systematically reinforced. This is partly because by definition, generalization is an unreinforced (albeit declining) rate of responses. In describing training and probe sequence, it was suggested in Chapter 5 that responses given to probe items should not be reinforced. That suggestion was made because initially the clinician wishes to assess generalization. Since a probe is designed to find out the extent of generalization, if any, correct responses given to probe items should not be reinforced. However, within the context of maintenance, generalized responses, first documented through unreinforced probes, should be reinforced.

A target behavior that generalizes to the home situation can be reinforced by the family members. In such cases, the family members do not have the problem of initiating the behavior at home in order to reinforce it. In this sense, when stimulus generalization, response generalization, or both take place, it is not the end of programming efforts. It is the beginning of a maintenance strategy in natural environments.

The clinician, too, can reinforce generalized responses while not assessing them. When the client is taken to nonclinical situations such as stores and other public places, appropriate responses can be reinforced on a relatively large ratio (Hegde and McConn, 1981). Even in clinical situations, novel (untrained) responses can be required and reinforced (Goetz and Baer, 1973).

When generalized responses are reinforced, it is inappropriate to call it a "strategy to promote generalization." Technically, reinforced responses are not generalized responses. Generalized responses are reinforced precisely because generalization is not an enduring process. Unless generalized responses are quickly brought under the control of contingencies, there is no response maintenance. Therefore, reinforcement of generalized responses should be considered a maintenance strategy.

HOLD INFORMAL TRAINING
SESSIONS IN NATURAL ENVIRONMENTS

Even before parents or others are asked to manage contingencies at home and in other situations, it may be worthwhile to hold some informal training sessions in those situations. As a result, the target behaviors are more likely to be produced in those extraclinical situations. Natural contingencies can then take over response maintenance.

Training sessions held in home and other nonclinical situations can use the "incidental" or in vivo teaching procedures (Hart and

Risley, 1975, 1980). These procedures are less formal than the discrete trial-based technique described in earlier chapters. In incidental teaching, stimuli and responses are allowed to vary as they do in real life situations. The clinician and the client might interact in typical manners in the client's home, stores, restaurants, playgrounds, and other places. Whenever the client produces the trained behaviors, the clinician might reinforce it, but the opportunities for such productions are not strictly controlled by the clinician. In essence, naturally occurring responses in real life situations may be reinforced. For example, a stutterer's fluent speech while ordering in a restaurant may be reinforced by the clinician. A child's correct production of targeted speech sounds or grammatic features in natural conversational speech may be reinforced at home. A deaf individual's correct sign language may be reinforced in a store.

It is important to hold informal training sessions in those situations where trained responses are not produced on the basis of generalization. It is also important to have parents or other family members present during such training so that they can eventually take over the response control function. Holding informal training sessions in situations that do not show generalization has been called sequential modification (Stokes and Baer, 1977).

Contingency management in natural settings such as stores and restaurants must be as subtle as it can be. A subtle signal such as a certain type of hand or finger movement can suggest to the client that the response was correct. A different signal might suggest that the target response was missed. The clinician and the client should agree beforehand on the meaning of such gestures.

TEACH SELF-CONTROL PROCEDURES

Probably one of the most effective maintenance strategies is to make the client his or her own therapist. Self-control is evident when a client is able to monitor his or her responses in such a way as to decrease or increase those responses. A client who can do this can maintain therapeutic gains with sporadic reinforcement from other persons. In recent years, a number of studies have been published in the behavioral self-control or self-management procedures (Gajar, Schloss, Schloss, and Thompson, 1984; O'Leary and Dubey, 1979; Rhode, Morgan, and Young, 1983; Rosenbaum and Drabman, 1979; Stevenson and Fantuzzo, 1984).

With behavioral analysis, self-control is not a mentalistic phenomenon. Self-control refers to certain kinds of responses that can be taught and learned. A person who hides cookies so that they are not readily available for indiscriminate consumption is showing self-control. A student who makes a practice of reading a certain number of pages in textbooks before being able to go to a movie also illustrates self-control. Similarly, a smoker who begins to closely monitor the number of cigarettes smoked per day in order to reduce smoking is modifying his or her own behavior through self-control. The stutterer who is able to measure his or her own dysfluencies reliably may be better able to control them. Clients who can plot their own incorrect phoneme productions may be better able to monitor their correct and incorrect productions of phonemes.

Whenever clients themselves indicate that their behavior did not meet the criterion or was simply incorrect, the clinician might reinforce such self-monitoring skills. Clients may be asked to mark the correct and incorrect responses on a separate recording sheet. They may also be taught to pause as soon as they exhibit a wrong response. This is self-administered timeout.

TEACH CONTINGENCY PRIMING

In spite of a clinician's best efforts to teach contingency management to significant others, sometimes they may fail to notice the production of target behaviors. In that case, the client would not be reinforced. One way of handling this problem is to teach the client to prime others to reinforce when he or she does produce clinically trained behaviors. In contingency priming, the client is taught certain actions that prompt other persons to reinforce him or her (Seymour and Stokes, 1976; Stokes, Fowler, and Baer, 1978).

Everyday examples of contingency priming are numerous. A child who writes something, shows it to the mother, and says "see, Mom, how nice is my handwriting" is priming reinforcement. Adults who draw attention to their good work and then ask questions like "how about this now?" are also priming reinforcement. Clinically, clients may be taught to draw other persons' attention to their own target responses in an effort to obtain reinforcers that may not otherwise be forthcoming. A stutterer who is now fluent as a result of therapy may specifically point out the fact that he or she is speaking fluently to the ignoring family members or colleagues. A child who has been taught to produce certain grammatic features may also be taught to draw the teacher's attention whenever those features are produced. In addition, the clients may also be asked to request their family or friends to signal the production of inappropriate behaviors. A client who is learning to speak without pitch breaks may ask his or her roommate to signal every time a pitch break is heard.

MAKE SURE THE
DURATION OF TREATMENT IS ADEQUATE

Sometimes the treatment gains may not be maintained simply because the duration of treatment was not adequate (Kazdin, 1984). Unless target behaviors are well established and stabilized, they may not be produced often enough in natural environments to be reinforced. As a result, target behaviors would not come under the influence of maintaining contingencies.

The clinician must make sure that the trained behaviors are occurring reliably in extraclinical situations either on the basis of generalization or because of the influence of maintaining contingencies. Periodic probes in extraclinical situations will help determine whether target behaviors are produced in those situations and, if so, to what extent. An extremely low response rate in everyday situations might in some cases suggest that more treatment is needed. A premature termination of the treatment program or a premature introduction of a maintenance strategy may both be detrimental to response maintenance.

FOLLOW UP AND ARRANGE
FOR BOOSTER TREATMENT

Booster treatment is that treatment given some time after the client is dismissed from the original program. Many clients can benefit from a booster treatment program. There is not much empirical evidence regarding the need for booster treatment across different disorders. Clinical impressions suggest that the need for booster treatment probably varies from disorder to disorder. For example, most stutterers can benefit from, and some absolutely need, booster treatment.

The need for booster treatment is typically established through follow-up procedures. Unfortunately, follow-up procedures are one of the most neglected aspects of treatment in communicative disorders. Very few follow-up studies are published in the specialty's journal. The clinician must establish a regular follow-up procedure in which dismissed clients are periodically recalled to the clinic. The purpose is to measure response maintenance over time.

A follow-up is nothing but a probe of previously trained target behaviors. The behaviors must be sampled adequately at the level of conversational speech. A conversational speech sample of extended duration is needed to calculate the percent correct response rate. When appropriate, oral reading samples, telephone conversations, and conversation with unfamiliar people may also be sampled. These latter procedures are especially important in a follow-up of treated stutterers. In addition, clients, parents, or both may be asked to tape conversational speech samples at home and send them to the clinician on a periodic basis. They may be requested to bring two or more recorded samples to the clinic when they come for a follow-up.

In order to establish reliability, a minimum of two samples of each speech task must be obtained. The results are analyzed the same way as any assessment or probe data. The most important factor is the measured rate of target responses across samples. If the rate of response has fallen below the set criterion, then there is a need for booster treatment.

Typically, booster treatment is not as extensive or intensive as the original treatment. Often a session or two may be sufficient to reinstate the rate of response recorded at the time of the original dismissal. A greater number of treatment sessions may be needed if deterioration in response rate has been severe. Even then, most clients recover their target behaviors fairly rapidly under booster treatment sessions.

Booster treatment may consist of the same treatment given originally, or it may be a variation of it. Entirely new treatment procedures can also be used during booster sessions, although in this case the eventual response maintenance cannot be attributed to any one treatment.

The first follow-up after the initial dismissal of the client may be scheduled after three months. Assuming that the target behaviors are maintained, the next follow-up may be scheduled after six months. Subsequent follow-ups may be done on an annual basis. Any time a follow-up measure shows a deterioration in response rate, booster treatment is arranged. After a booster treatment, a more frequent follow-up may be required until it is established that the target behaviors are maintained. In other words, the first follow-up subsequent to booster treatment may be arranged after three months.

At the time of dismissal, clients or parents must be informed that they should get in touch with the clinic any time they see a change for the worse in treated behaviors. This can help initiate needed booster treatment before a scheduled follow-up takes place.

SUMMARY

Discrimination and generalization are two concepts that are especially relevant to an analysis and training of language behaviors. Discrimination involves different responses to different stimuli. It is achieved through a process called differential reinforcement. Whenever there is unacceptable generalization, discrimination training is needed.

Generalization is a declining response rate under changing stimulus and response properties in the absence of reinforcement. As such, it should not be the final goal of clinical intervention. However, before it becomes extinguished, a generalized response rate can serve as a basis for maintenance strategies. Stimulus and response generalization are the two major types of generalization and each has a variety of subtypes. To the extent that generalization can serve as a basis for maintenance strategies, it is desirable to take steps to promote its occurrence.

The final criterion of treatment success is response maintenance in everyday situations. Response maintenance refers to durability of treated behaviors across situations and persons and over time. Responses are maintained not because they show an initial (and temporary) generalization but because they come under natural maintaining contingencies. All contingencies, including those that occur naturally, have stimulus, response, and consequence variables. Therefore, maintenance strategies instituted by clinicians must take into consideration these three aspects of the behavioral contingency.

In promoting an initial generalization and subsequent maintenance of target behaviors, the clinician can take several steps. Strategies of maintenance must be thought of even before treatment is begun. The strategies can be conceptualized in terms of (1) stimulus manipulations, (2) response considerations, and (3) consequence manipulations.

Stimulus manipulations include (1) selecting standard stimuli from the client's natural environment, (2) selecting common verbal antecedents, (3) varying audience antecedents, and (4) varying physical setting controls.

Response considerations include (1) selecting client-specific target behaviors, (2) selecting multiple exemplars of each of the target behaviors, and (3) reinforcing complex response topographies.

Consequence manipulations include (1) using intermittent reinforcement schedules, (2) using conditioned reinforcers, (3) delaying reinforcement, (4) training significant others, (5) reinforcing generalized responses, (6) holding informal training sessions in natural settings, (7) teaching the client self-control procedures, (8) teaching the client contingency priming, (9) providing treatment for an appropriate duration, and (10) arranging for follow-up and booster treatment.

There is an urgent need to experimentally demonstrate the effectiveness of these and other maintenance strategies. It is hoped that since clinicians are now more concerned about maintenance than ever before, systematic research information on better sets of maintenance techniques will become available in the near future.

STUDY GUIDE

Answer the following questions in technical language. Check your answers with the text. When necessary, rewrite your answers.

1. Define discrimination.
2. State the clinical need for discrimination training.
3. What is differential reinforcement?
4. What are concepts?
5. What is abstraction in behavioral analysis?
6. How do you compare and contrast generalization and discrimination?
7. Define generalization.
8. Define stimulus generalization.
9. What is a generalization gradient?
10. Summarize the basic research information on stimulus generalization.
11. Define the following types of stimulus generalization:
    a. Physical stimulus generalization.
    b. Verbal stimulus generalization.
    c. Physical setting generalization.
    d. Audience generalization.
    e. Factorial stimulus generalization.
12. Write your own examples of each type of stimulus generalization.
13. Define and describe response generalization.
14. Write your own examples of response generalization.
15. What is intraverbal generalization? Give examples.
16. Describe response mode generalization.
17. How is "comprehension" treated in behavioral analysis?
18. Describe concurrent stimulus-response generalization.
19. State precisely why generalization should not be the final goal of clinical intervention programs.
20. State the two problems that emerge when generalization is treated as the final goal of treatment.
21. State why "programming generalization" is conceptually confusing.
22. What is the final goal of clinical treatment?
23. How are responses maintained?

24. What are the three sets of maintenance strategies?
25. Define and describe each of the specific maintenance strategies. Give examples.
26. What are the four stimulus manipulations related to response maintenance strategies?
27. How do you vary physical setting controls?
28. Why should you reinforce complex response topographies?
29. How can you determine how many exemplars should be trained?
30. When and why do you use intermittent reinforcement schedules?
31. What additional steps do you take while using primary reinforcers?
32. What do you mean by "train significant others"?
33. What do you mean by "shift the locus of control"?
34. As a maintenance strategy, can you reinforce generalized responses?
35. Is reinforcing generalized responses a "strategy to promote generalization"? Justify your answer.
36. How do you manage contingencies while holding informal training sessions in naturalistic settings?
37. Define self-control.
38. What are some of the self-control procedures you can use?
39. What is contingency priming?
40. How is treatment duration related to maintenance?
41. What is the purpose of a follow-up?
42. How do you measure behaviors during a follow-up?
43. What is "booster treatment"? When is it appropriate?

REFERENCES

Carr, E. G., and Kologinsky, E. (1983). Acquisition of sign language by autistic children. II: Spontaneity and generalization effects. *Journal of Applied Behavior Analysis, 16,* 297–314.

Colletti, G., and Harris, S. L. (1977). Behavior modification in the home: Siblings as behavior modifiers, parents as observers. *Journal of Abnormal Child Psychology, 5,* 21–30.

Connell, P., and McReynolds, L. V. (1981). An experimental analysis of children's generalization during lexical learning: Comprehension or production. *Applied Psycholinguistics, 2,* 309–332.

Costello, J. M. (1983). Generalization across settings. In J. Miller, D. Yoder, and R. Schiefelbusch (Eds.), *Contemporary issues in language intervention.* Rockville, MD: ASHA Reports No. 12.

Dale, P. S. (1976). *Language development: Structure and function.* New York: Holt, Rinehart and Winston.

Drabman, R. S., Hammer, D., and Rosenbaum, M. S. (1979). Assessing generalization in behavior modification with children: The generalization map. *Behavioral Assessment, 1,* 203–204.

Duker, P. C., and Morsink, H. (1984). Acquisition and cross-setting generalization of manual signs with severely retarded individuals. *Journal of Applied Behavior Analysis, 17,* 93–103.

Faw, G. D., Reid, D. H., Schepis, M. M., Fitzgerald, J. R., and Welty, P. A., (1981). Involving institutional staff in the development and maintenance of sign language skills with profoundly retarded persons. *Journal of Applied Behavior Analysis, 14,* 411–423.

Ferster, C. B., Culbertson, S., and Boren, M. C. P. (1975). *Behavior principles* (2nd ed.). Englewood Cliffs, NJ: Prentice-Hall.

Gajar, A., Schloss, P. J., Schloss, C. N., and Thompson, C. K. (1984). Effects of feedback and self-monitoring on head trauma youths' conversation skills. *Journal of Applied Behavior Analysis, 17,* 353–358.

Goetz, E. M., and Baer, D. M. (1973). Social control of form diversity and the emergence of new forms in children's blockbuilding. *Journal of Applied Behavior Analysis, 6,* 105–113.

Graziano, A. M. (1978). Parents as behavior therapists. In M. Hersen, R. M. Eisler, and P. M. Miller (Eds.), *Progress in behavior modification: Vol. 4.* New York: Academic Press.

Guess, D., and Baer, D. M. (1973). Some experimental analyses of linguistic development in institutionalized retarded children. In B. B. Lahey, (Ed.), *Modification of language behavior* (pp. 3–60). Springfield, IL: Charles C Thomas.

Handleman, J. S. (1979). Generalization by autistic-type children of verbal responses across settings. *Journal of Applied Behavior Analysis, 12,* 273–282.

Hart, B. M., and Risley, T. R. (1975). Incidental teaching of language in the preschool. *Journal of Applied Behavior Analysis, 8,* 411–420.

Hart, B. M. and Risley, T. R. (1980). In vivo language intervention: Unanticipated general effects. *Journal of Applied Behavior Analysis, 13,* 407–437.

Hegde, M. N. (1980). An experimental-clinical analysis of grammatical and behavioral distinctions between verbal auxiliary and copula. *Journal of Speech and Hearing Research, 23,* 864–877.

Hegde, M. N., and Gierut, J. (1979). The operant training and generalization of pronouns and a verb form in a language delayed child. *Journal of Communication Disorders, 12,* 23–34.

Hegde, M. N., and McConn, J. (1981). Language training: Some data on response classes and generalization to an occupational setting. *Journal of Speech and Hearing Disorders, 46,* 353–358.

Hegde, M. N., Noll, M. J., and Pecora, R. (1979). A study of some factors affecting generalization of language training. *Journal of Speech and Hearing Disorders, 44,* 301–320.

Ingham, R. J. (1984). Generalization and maintenance of treatment. In R. F. Curlee and W. H. Perkins (Eds.), *Nature and treatment of stuttering: New directions* (pp. 447–471). San Diego: College-Hill Press.

Kalish, H. I. (1981). *From behavioral science to behavior modification.* New York: McGraw-Hill.

Kazdin, A. E. (1984). *Behavior modification in applied settings* (3rd ed.). Homewood, IL: Dorsey Press.

Kazdin, A. E., and Polster, R. (1973). Intermittent token reinforcement and response maintenance in extinction. *Behavior Therapy, 4,* 386–391.

Keller, M., and Bucher, B. (1979). Transfer between receptive and productive language in developmentally disabled children. *Journal of Applied Behavior Analysis, 12,* 311.

Koegel, R. L., Glahn, T. J., and Nieminen, G. S. (1978). Generalization of parent training results. *Journal of Applied Behavior Analysis, 11,* 95–109.

Lovaas, I. O., Koegel, R. L., Simmons, J., and Stevens-Long, J. (1973). Some generalization and follow-up measures on autistic children in behavior therapy. *Journal of Applied Behavior Analysis, 6,* 131–166.

Marholin D., II, Siegel, L. J., and Phillips, D. (1976). Treatment and transfer: A search for empirical procedures. In M. Hersen, R. M. Eisler, and P. M. Miller (Eds.), *Progress in behavior modification* (Vol. 3) (pp. 294–342). New York: Academic Press.

McGee, G. G., Krantz, P. J., Mason, D., and McClannahan, L. E. (1983). A modified incidental teaching procedure for autistic youth: Acquisition and generalization of receptive object labels. *Journal of Applied Behavior Analysis, 16,* 329–338.

O'Dell, S. (1974). Training parents in behavior modification: A review. *Psychological Bulletin, 81,* 418–433.

O'Leary, S. G., and Dubey, D. R. (1979). Applications of self-control procedures by children: A review. *Journal of Applied Behavior Analysis, 12,* 449–465.

Owens, R. E., Jr. (1984). *Language development: An introduction.* Columbus, OH: Charles E. Merrill.

Rhode, G., Morgan, D. P., and Young, K. R. (1983). Generalization and maintenance of treatment gains of behaviorally handicapped students from resource rooms to regular classrooms using self-evaluation procedures. *Journal of Applied Behavior Analysis, 16,* 171–188.

Rincover, A., and Koegel, R. L. (1975). Setting generality and stimulus control in autistic children. *Journal of Applied Behavior Analysis, 8,* 235–246.

Rosenbaum, M. S., and Drabman, R. S. (1979). Self-control training in the classroom: A review and critique. *Journal of Applied Behavior Analysis, 12,* 467–485.

Scott, R. R., Himadi, W., and Keane, T. (1983). A review of generalization in social skills training: Suggestions for future research. In M. Hersen, R. M. Eisler, and P. M. Miller (Eds.), *Progress in behavior modification* (Vol. 15) (pp. 114–172). New York: Academic Press.

Schumaker, J. B., and Sherman, J. A. (1978). Parents as intervention agents. In R. L. Schiefelbusch (Ed.), *Language intervention strategies* (pp. 237–326). Baltimore: University Park Press.

Seymour, F. W., and Stokes, T. F. (1976). Self-recording in training girls to increase work and evoke staff praise in an institution for offenders. *Journal of Applied Behavior Analysis, 9,* 41–54.

Skinner, B. F. (1953). *Science and human behavior.* New York: Macmillan.

Skinner, B. F. (1969). *Contingencies of reinforcement: A theoretical analysis.* New York: Appleton-Century-Crofts.

Skinner, B. F. (1974). *About behaviorism.* New York: Vintage Books.

Stevenson, H. C., and Fantuzzo, J. W. (1984). Application of the "generalization map" to self-control intervention with school-aged children. *Journal of Applied Behavior Analysis, 17,* 203–212.

Stokes, T. F., and Baer, D. M. (1977). An implicit technology of generalization. *Journal of Applied Behavior Analysis, 10,* 349–367.

Stokes, T. F., Fowler, S., and Baer, D. M. (1978). Training preschool children to recruit natural communities of reinforcement. *Journal of Applied Behavior Analysis, 11,* 285–303.

Welch, S. J., and Pear, J. J. (1980). Generalization of naming responses to objects in the natural environment as a function of training stimulus modality with retarded children. *Journal of Applied Behavior Analysis, 13,* 629–643.

Williams, G. C., and McReynolds, L. V. (1976). The relationship between discrimination and articulation training in children with misarticulation. *Journal of Speech and Hearing Research, 18,* 401–412.

Winokur, S. (1976). *A primer of verbal behavior: An operant view.* Englewood Cliffs, NJ: Prentice-Hall.

Chapter 8

Decreasing Undesirable Behaviors

So far, techniques designed to increase behaviors that exist at a low level of frequency have been described, as well as techniques for shaping new behaviors and those that support response maintenance.

In Chapter 8, the following points will be described:

- Procedures designed to decrease undesirable and interfering behaviors
- Extinction: the concept and procedures
- Punishment: the concept and procedures
- Type I punishment
- Type II punishment
- Type III punishment
- Additional effects of punishment
- How to program punishing contingencies

It was pointed out in Chapter 4 that the two most important tasks of speech and language pathologists are to (1) increase desirable target behaviors and (2) decrease the undesirable behaviors of their clients. The procedures described in the previous chapters, including positive and negative reinforcement, shaping, modeling, and differential reinforcement help achieve the first task. This chapter is concerned with the second basic task of speech-language clinicians.

Generally speaking, clients can exhibit two sets of behaviors that need to be decreased. The first set of behaviors are those that are incompatible with the desirable target behaviors. The second set are those that interfere with the training process.

Incompatible behaviors are the typical wrong responses clients give in place of appropriate responses. Misarticulated sounds, stutterings, inappropriate pitch, and the wrong usage of grammatic features are among the behaviors that are incompatible with the desirable communicative behaviors. A misarticulated speech sound is incompatible with the correct production of the same speech sound. Similarly, stutterings are incompatible with fluency.

The second set of behaviors, more than being incompatible with the desirable communicative behaviors, interfere with the treatment process. A client who does not pay attention to the stimulus, a child who cries and whines in the sessions, a teenage stutterer who yawns incessantly during the treatment, or children who begin to play with the material on hand all illustrate interfering behaviors. Also, most uncooperative behaviors, such as wiggling in the chair, off-seat behaviors, interruptive talking, lying under the table, constantly paying attention to irrelevant stimuli in therapy rooms, constitute interfering behaviors. Unless these behaviors are eliminated or reduced, the clinician cannot focus upon the desirable target behaviors. Therefore, control of these behaviors becomes a priority.

Throughout this chapter, the term undesirable behaviors will be used to include both the types of responses that need to be reduced. Whenever more specificity is needed, the term incompatible responses or interfering responses will be used.

There are two sets of techniques for decreasing undesirable behaviors: extinction and punishment.

EXTINCTION

Like most techniques of behavior change, the phenomenon of extinction was originally formulated in the context of laboratory experiments in both the Pavlovian (classical) and Skinnerian (operant) conditioning. The term extinction refers to the procedure of terminating the reinforcer for a response (Ferster, Culbertson, and Boren, 1975; Holland and Skinner, 1961; Kazdin, 1984). If the response is continuously evoked without reinforcement, the response rate eventually decreases and may even reach zero. Extinction is common to both classical and operant responses. The Pavlovian dog will stop salivating if the experimenter continues to present the bell without food. The Skinnerian pigeon will in due course stop pecking the button when that response no longer produces food.

It is important to realize that extinction refers to a behavioral procedure that produces certain changes in the response rate. When a previously reinforced response no longer produces reinforcers, the subject will not stop responding abruptly. In fact, the subject may redouble the efforts and increase the rate of response, presumably to produce the reinforcer. But if the responses continue to go unreinforced, the rate will eventually decrease to its prereinforcement level. The rate of decrease is typically slow. As such, extinction is a gradual, not a sudden, process. Since an initial increase in responses can occur when the reinforcer is withheld, it is not appropriate to define extinction as a decrease in the rate of response under no reinforcement.

Generally speaking, the concept of extinction is similar to what people call ignoring. When an action is consistently ignored by a person, then that action becomes less likely in the presence of that person. The term extinction captures this process in a scientific and systematic manner.

Factors that Affect Extinction

How soon a response will be extinguished after its reinforcer has been withheld depends upon a number of factors. The first, and probably the most important, is the reinforcement schedule on which the response was maintained before extinction was initiated. Extensive laboratory research has shown that behaviors maintained on an intermittent reinforcement schedule are more difficult to extinguish than those maintained on a continuous schedule (Ferster et al., 1979; Ferster and Skinner, 1957). Such behaviors persist even when the reinforcer is withdrawn. The relatively long duration it takes to extinguish the response may afford opportunities for unplanned reinforcement.

The second factor affecting extinction is the amount of reinforcement the response has earned in the past. A heavily reinforced response is more difficult to extinguish than the one reinforced not so heavily. The third factor is the duration for which the response has been reinforced. A response reinforced over a long period of time is more difficult to extinguish than the one reinforced for a shorter duration. The fourth factor is whether the response has ever been put under an extinction procedure. The response that has undergone some extinction trials before is easier to extinguish than the one being extinguished for the first time.

In essence, the most difficult response to extinguish is the one that has been reinforced intermittently, with large amounts of reinforcement, over a long period of time, and with no prior history of extinction.

Isolating the Reinforcer

Before extinction can be initiated, the reinforcer that is maintaining the response must be identified. This is not a major problem in laboratory research. The experimenter will have first conditioned the response with a specific reinforcer, which is then withheld, and the subject is allowed to respond. On the other hand, in clinical situations, we typically do not know the conditioning history of a given client's undesirable behaviors. Nevertheless, the procedure of extinction requires that specific reinforcers for those responses be withheld. Therefore, the clinician often has to guess at the possible reinforcers maintaining given undesirable behaviors and then withhold them. This is the reason why extinction is less efficient in clinical situations than in the laboratory experiments.

In isolating potential reinforcers of undesirable behaviors, the clinician depends upon past research. It is generally known that most undesirable behaviors are maintained by social attention (Kazdin, 1984; Whaley and Malott, 1970). A complete withdrawal of attention can decrease many undesirable behaviors. Unfortunately, some clinicians continue to pay attention even when the child is crying, whining, or lying under the table. When the client interrupts the training trials by asking irrelevant questions or by narrating "you know what" types of stories, clinicians might reinforce by paying attention and responding in typical manners. At other times, clinicians try to talk the child out of interfering behaviors. But this very effort on the part of a clinician may be the reinforcing event maintaining such undesirable responses.

In many clinical situations, the extinction procedure can be somewhat uncomfortable to the clinician. When a child begins to cry in a session, the clinician must cease all forms of attention and must turn away from the child. The clinician should not be doing anything (such as reorganizing the stimulus material) that might be reinforcing to the child. The crying behavior may not subside immediately. Only when the clinican persists with the extinction procedure will there be a decrease in crying behavior.

The possibility of an initial increase in the response rate under the extinction procedure should be handled very carefully. Sometimes, the clinician might get concerned about this increase and do something that will actually reinforce the response. For example, when the intensity of the crying behavior increases, the clinician might pick up the child, or bring the mother into the therapy room. It is very important for the clinician to resist the temptation to stop that behavior by other means at this time.

It is necessary to make sure that a client on an extinction schedule is not receiving reinforcement. A child lying under the table in a treatment session may be looking at a comic book or playing with a small toy. In this case, even though the clinician withdraws attention, the response did not come under extinction. In everyday situations, when one person is trying to ignore a behavior, another person may be reinforcing it. In modifying child behaviors, parents must make sure that they are consistent in applying the same contingency.

Although in many cases reinforcers maintaining responses are difficult to identify, the interfering behaviors children show in most clinical situations can be effectively controlled by a systematic use of attention. Such responses as "is it time to go yet?" "we are all done for today" and "you know what?" are best ignored. If the child begins to play with some of the stimulus materials or reinforcers, they should be promptly removed from the subject's reach. If the child looks at the mirror and makes faces, the seating arrangement can be changed so that the child does not face the mirror. These examples illustrate how reinforcers can be withdrawn in order to extinguish inappropriate responses.

Combination of Extinction and Reinforcement

Typically, undesirable behaviors take the place of desirable behaviors. Therefore, it is often useful to keep the desirable behavior also targeted while scheduling extinction for undesirable behaviors. This means that the clinician must combine positive reinforcement for desirable behaviors and extinction for undesirable behaviors. This way, while a competing response is being weakened, an alternative response is being strengthened. It is known that extinction of a response is faster when an alternative response is positively reinforced (Sundel and Sundel, 1975).

To use the earlier example, crying behavior may be put on extinction. While crying is being extinguished, the clinician should be alert to any desirable changes in that behavior. Even a brief period of no crying should be immediately reinforced. While nonattending behavior is being ignored, attending behavior must be positively reinforced. Sometimes clinicians make the mistake of not taking note of the alternative behavior quickly enough, with the result that the undesirable behavior picks up speed again.

Limitations of Extinction

Some experiments have shown that extinction may have certain negative side effects. When the reinforcer is withheld, reactions of anger, frustration, and even aggression may be shown by the client. The author once observed a child whose crying behavior under extinction was interrupted by shouts such as "I don't like you" and "you are not nice." In everyday situations, adults too show emotional reactions when the reinforcer is not forthcoming. A flat tire might force the driver to curse and kick the car, and a losing tennis star might throw his racket on the ground.

The best way of handling these emotional reactions is to make sure that desirable behaviors are always identified prior to the initiation of extinction, and then even the earliest signs of those behaviors are reinforced. The actual extinction and reinforcement contingency must be made clear to the client. For example, the clinician might tell a crying child that as soon as he or she stops crying, they can go out to see the mother.

Another problem with extinction is that the extinguished response may recover sooner or later. If the response is reinforced at this time, it might rebound with remarkable force. However, if that behavior is put back on extinction, the process will be quicker than originally. With succeeding cycles of extinction, the behavior is eliminated sooner and with more lasting effects.

Extinction may not be a method of choice under some circumstances, however. When the undesirable behavior is aggressive, self-destructive, or highly disruptive, extinction may not be the best strategy. Since extinction is a slow process, aggressive behaviors might result in damage to other persons or property. Before they are extinguished, self-destructive behaviors can cause considerable harm to the person. Extremely disruptive behaviors in clinic and classroom situations may have to be controlled by other means that produce faster results.

Carefully planned extinction schedules combined with positive reinforcement can be very effective in controlling undesirable behaviors while at the same time encouraging desirable alternative responses. Once extinction is initiated, the clinician must make sure that the client will not be reinforced until signs of desirable behaviors occur.

PUNISHMENT

Punishment is another set of techniques that can decrease undesirable behaviors. Some clinicians may be alarmed at this term, but it is not used in the popular sense here. In everyday use, the term is emotionally charged and the popular use of punishment is often questionable.

Punishment refers to a scientific principle and certain procedures based upon that principle. There are both laboratory and applied research data supporting the practice of punishment techniques when they are warranted. A wide variety of basic and applied research has pointed out the strengths and limitations of punishment, along with the best possible ways of using the procedures in clinical settings (Axelrod and Apsche, 1983; Matson and DiLorenzo, 1984).

Definition of Punishment

There are three types of punishment, which will be defined separately. However, a general definition of punishment as a principle and as a set of procedures can be offered here. As a principle, it states that certain empirical operations are associated with a reduction in response rates. As a procedure, punishment can be defined as a set of objective procedures that, when made contingent upon a response, will decrease the rate of that response.

It should be noted that the definition of punishment does not include any reference to emotional states, subjective feelings, pain, or how the person receiving punishment evaluates it. The definition focuses upon rates of responses. A stimulus consequence that reduces a response rate is a punisher. Popularly, punishment is often thought of as the presentation of something unpleasant or painful. In this case, the rate of the response for which unpleasant stimuli were intended is ignored. In behavioral science, punishment is defined solely on the basis of what happens to the rate of responses on which the contingency is placed. As you know, positive reinforcers are also defined exclusively on the basis of their effects upon response rates.

How the stimulus is evaluated by the person who delivers the punishing stimulus is also irrelevant to the definition of punishment. A clinician may think that some stimulus such as a verbal "no" ought to be a punisher because he or she feels that it is unpleasant. However, the response on which it has been made contingent may or may not decrease. What is important is the effect of the stimulus on the observable response rate, not its presumed property or predicted effects.

What is physically painful or psychologically aversive may or may not act as a punisher. Parents may shout at the child in order to reduce a particular behavior, but they soon find out that shouting does not help. If they did not realize this, they will be shouting louder and louder with no effect, and this too happens quite often. Parents know that even spanking may not reduce behaviors for which it has been used. Verbal statements such as "you are wrong" may or may not act as punishers, even though most people find them to be unpleasant. Therefore, it is important to define effects of stimuli only when those effects upon some behavior are actually demonstrated.

There exists a potential confusion between negative reinforcement and punishment. Some people use the term negative reinforcement instead of punishment. As you recall from Chapter 4, negative reinforcement is by definition a reinforcement procedure. It increases rates of responses. Punishment, on the other hand, decreases response rates. Since the two procedures have opposite effects on behavior, they should not be confused.

Type I Punishment

Type I punishment is the reduction in a response rate produced by the contingent presentation of stimulus events. Although stimulus presentations are referred to, it should be noted that in this particular context, they are not antecedents but consequences of responses. A certain stimulus event is presented soon after the response is made, and as a result, there is a reduction in the rate of responses. This is then classified as Type I punishment.

A variety of stimulus consequences have been made contingent upon responses in Type I punishment (Matson and DiLorenzo, 1984). In many laboratory experiments, electric shock has been used. Shock has been used on an experimental basis in treating a variety of behavior disorders. It has been used most frequently in the treatment of highly disruptive, aggressive, and self-stimulatory behaviors that were difficult to control by other means. Many investigators who have used shock as a form of punishment have justified it on the basis that the untreated undesirable behaviors, such as violent self-stimulatory behaviors and persistent vomiting, would have caused more damage to the patient. Nevertheless, the use of electric shock has declined in recent years, and other types of consequences have replaced shock.

In the field of communicative disorders, the effects of shock on stuttering have been experimentally evaluated in a number of studies (Ingham, 1984; Siegel, 1970). The purpose of this research has been to find out if stuttering behaviors are affected by their consequences. The majority of studies have shown that stuttering behaviors decrease under contingent electric shock, although the magnitude of the reduction has not been of clinical significance. A few studies have also reported an increase in stuttering when the subject is stimulated with shock (Hegde, 1985; Martin, St. Louis, Haroldson, and Hasbrouck, 1975). Increase in response rates under known punishment procedures is a well-documented phenomenon. It is described in a later section.

Mechanically generated noise has also been a stimulus used in Type I punishment. It is known that noise, when made contingent upon specified responses, can reduce their rate. Typically, a short burst of noise is delivered through headphones. In communicative disorders, the experimental and clinical effects of noise on stuttering has been evaluated most extensively (Hegde, 1985; Ingham, 1984). Response contingent noise is known to decrease stuttering dramatically. Unfortunately, the effects do not seem to last.

There are some studies in which noise is presented continuously while the stutterer is talking. This can also reduce stuttering, but it must be realized that this is not a punishment procedure, since there is no response-contingent presentation of noise. Continuous presentation of noise is described as a masking procedure.

Probably the most common of the Type I punishing stimuli are verbal. Verbal responses such as "no," "wrong," "not correct," "I do not agree," and "that is not true" can have punishing effects on responses. Verbal stimuli are also probably the most socially acceptable of the punishing stimuli. They may have fewer negative effects, and their use is extensive in natural environments.

Except in the field of stuttering, there are not many studies in which the use of verbal punishment has been tested. A few studies involving stuttering have shown that verbal stimuli such as "wrong" can be a punisher (Siegel, 1970). However, there are no stuttering treatment procedures based exclusively on verbal (or other) punishment procedure. In fact, it is true of the treatment of all kinds of communicative disorders. Typically, punishing verbal stimuli are a part of total treatment programs that include positive reinforcement procedures designed to increase desirable behaviors. In the treatment of most communicative disorders, clinicians usually say "no," "wrong," or "not correct" whenever incorrect responses are produced by the client, while reinforcing correct responses with verbal praise or other kinds of reinforcers.

There are other kinds of Type I punishing stimuli. Some are called noxious substances, which are not physically harmful but can reduce the rate of responses when presented contingently. From a subjective standpoint, noxious stimuli are unpleasant to either smell, hear, or taste, and therefore persons try to avoid them. Ammonia capsules and 100 percent lemon juice, among other substances, have been used as punishers in some studies. As the use of electric shock declined, the use of noxious substances apparently increased (Matson and DiLorenzo, 1984).

Whether noise, shock, or verbal "no," Type I punishing stimuli are presented immediately after a specified response is made. In order to be effective, the selected stimulus must be presented at full strength and on a continuous schedule. Used appropriately, Type I punishment can be extremely useful in controlling a variety of undesirable behaviors in clinical settings.

Type II Punishment

Unlike Type I punishment, in which a stimulus is presented response contingently, Type II punishment involves a contingent withdrawal of some event. Type II punishment can be defined as a response contingent withdrawal of reinforcers or reinforcing state of affairs resulting in a decreased rate of that response.

There are two major procedures under Type II punishment. The variations come about because of what is withdrawn response contingently and how it is done. The two distinct procedures are timeout and response cost. These procedures have been researched extensively and have been applied to a variety of behavioral and communicative disorders. By and large, the use of Type II punishment is less controversial, and generally very effective.

Timeout. Timeout (TO) actually means time out from positive reinforcement. It can be defined as a period of nonreinforcement imposed response contingently, resulting in a decreased rate of that response. This period of time can be imposed in different ways, giving rise to variations in TO procedures. There are three major types of TO (Brantner and Doherty, 1983).

The first and probably the most extreme form is called isolation TO. It involves the removal of the person from the environment and placing him or her in a specially designed situation with limited reinforcers. The parents may send a child to a barren room for a specified period of time. Timeout booths and prisons also illustrate this procedure. When a person is placed in a barren room or a TO booth, naturally occurring reinforcers are denied during the TO period. Prisons, on the other hand, may or may not act as punishers for a variety of reasons. Probably the most important reason is that the prison terms are not response contingent. Isolation TO is controversial and is used mostly in institutional settings with appropriate legal and ethical safeguards.

The second type is called exclusion TO. It is probably used more frequently in educational settings. A teacher might ask a misbehaving child to sit outside the classroom, in a corner, or facing the wall. The child in this case is excluded from the normal activities of the classroom but is not isolated. Exclusion TO is not used often in clinical speech-language services. When the sessions are as brief as they are in the treatment of communicative disorders, the punishment procedures must also be brief.

The third type is known as nonexclusion TO. In the most common form of nonexclusion TO, the client is simply given a response contingent signal, which initiates a brief period of TO during which (1) the clinician will not interact with the client, (2) the client is prohibited from responding, and hence (3) there will be no reinforcers forthcoming. This form of TO can be described as a "frozen moment" of no interaction. For example, any time a client gives a wrong response, the clinician might say "stop," and avoid the eye contact for a brief period, such as 5 seconds.

Nonexclusion TO is socially more acceptable than the other forms. It does not involve physical removal, isolation, or exclusion. This technique is known to be very effective in reducing a variety of incorrect and interfering behaviors (Brantner and Doherty, 1983). In clinical speech and language sessions, this type of TO has been used more frequently. Several studies have demonstrated the effectiveness of nonexclusion TO in the treatment of stuttering (Costello, 1975; James, 1981; Martin, Khul, and Haroldson, 1972; Parsons, 1984). The general procedure involves giving a signal such as "stop" contingent upon stuttering response and imposing a brief TO period during which the client is not allowed to talk and there is no eye contact with the clinician. As long as the stutterer is able to sustain fluent speech, the clinician continues to reinforce with such social reinforcers as eye contact, smile, and attention.

Nonexclusion TO can be effectively used in controlling various kinds of interfering behaviors exhibited by young clients during clinical sessions. Often, this type of TO may be combined with Type I punishment involving verbal punishers. For example, whenever a child yawns or looks away from the stimulus item, the clinician might say "no" and then avoid eye contact for a few seconds.

Response Cost. Response cost is a procedure in which specified reinforcers are withdrawn response contingently so that the rate of response decreases (Pazulinec, Meyerrose, and Sajwaj, 1983). Each incorrect response results in a loss of a reinforcer the person has access to. In other words, each wrong response costs the client a reinforcer.

The procedural distinction between TO and response cost must be clear. In TO, the person himself or herself may be removed from a reinforcing state of affairs. Or, the person is denied the opportunity to respond. In TO, a specific reinforcer is not taken away from the person in a response contingent manner. On the other hand, in response cost, each response results in the loss of a specified reinforcer. The person is neither removed from the scene nor prevented from responding. In everyday terms, the difference can be seen in terms of a prison term as against fines. While the prison term is supposed to act like TO, the fines are supposed to act like response cost. (However, neither the prison term nor the fines may be effective because of a lack of response contingency.)

The response cost procedure is relatively easy to use. It is not as restrictive as some forms of TO, and it may generate much less emotional resistance. It is known to be very effective in controlling a variety of interfering and inappropriate behaviors in many clinical, educational, and home settings (Pazulinec et al., 1983).

In order to implement the response cost procedure, the client must have accumulated a certain amount of reinforcers, or must at least have access to some reinforcers. Many clinicians reinforce the correct production of target behaviors by giving points, stickers, stars, tokens, and edible items that can be collected by the client. When there is a certain accumulation of these reinforcers, the clinician can initiate the response cost procedures to speed up the reduction of still troublesome incorrect responses, or to control interfering behaviors. Reinforcers earned for correct responses may be lost for incorrect ones. For example, in a language training study, Hegde and Gierut (1979) reinforced correct responses with a spoonful of cereal on an FR2 schedule but withdrew the same amount of cereal every time an incorrect response was made. Similarly, reinforcers can be lost as a result of interfering responses.

In some cases, the clients were given a certain number of tokens noncontingently (Pazulinec et al., 1983). That is, they did not have to earn the tokens that they could use to buy various necessities and privileges in institutional settings such as mental hospitals. Then throughout the day, the client behaviors were monitored. Every specified inappropriate behavior then resulted in a loss of a certain amount of tokens the clients already had. In this case, the tokens were not earned by the clients, but they lost them as a result of inappropriate behaviors. This variation can be used by the speech and language clinician by giving a certain number of tokens or points at the very beginning of a session, and taking them away as inappropriate behaviors are exhibited.

In some educational settings, response cost procedure can be arranged to reflect a group contingency. A certain number of points can be given to an entire class, and any inappropriate behavior on the part of any student can result in the loss of a point. Undesirable behaviors of groups are known to decrease under this arrangement.

In the treatment of communicative disorders, not many studies have experimentally evaluated the specific effects of response cost. A study by Halvorson (1971), however, has shown that response cost can be an effective procedure in the treatment of stuttering. In this study, when stutterers lost points on a counter every time they stuttered, the stuttering frequency decreased. In general, though, the technique is a part of an overall treatment strategy that typically includes reinforcement for desirable target behaviors. Every incorrect production of a phoneme or a grammatic morpheme may result in the loss of a reinforcer. Similarly, every time a client exhibits an interfering or uncooperative behavior, the clinician can withdraw a reinforcer earned by the client.

Type III Punishment

The third variety of punishment procedure requires the person to eliminate the effects of misbehavior and practice its counterpart, an appropriate behavior. This type of punishment is called overcorrection. There is some argument as to whether it is a variation of Type I punishment (Foxx and Bechtel, 1983), but for the sake of clarity, it is treated as a separate type in this book.

Overcorrection procedures were originally developed in the treatment of mental patients. They have been used mostly in institutional settings. Overcorrection has three components. The first requires the person to eliminate the immediate effects of a misbehavior, and the second, to vastly improve the environment. The third component requires that the person practice the incompatible, appropriate behavior again and again in the absence of reinforcement. For example, a patient who kicked a bucket of water and made a mess is first asked to straighten up the bucket and mop the floor. Second, the patient is required to mop and polish the floor of the entire ward. Third, the patient is asked to walk appropriately around the bucket several times (Matson and DiLorenzo, 1984).

The first two components are sometimes referred to as restitution, and the last component, positive practice. The restitution part requires not only that the effects of misbehavior are corrected but that the situation be improved beyond its original state. The positive practice part can be thought of as encouraging alternative, desirable behaviors, but it is still punishment because heavy work is made contingent upon misbehavior in the absence of positive reinforcement (Matson and DiLorenzo, 1984).

Overcorrection has been used extensively in a variety of settings to control a wide range of problem behaviors. In special educational settings, the technique is applicable in controlling disruptive and aggressive behaviors and in encouraging more appropriate social behaviors. An interesting example of the positive practice part of the overcorrection method can be found in a study by Barton and Osborne (1978). The authors increased the verbal sharing behavior, which was defined as either a verbal request to share another child's toys or an invitation to share one's own toys. The subjects were five hard of hearing children of kindergarten age. In a play situation, any occurrence of nonsharing behavior led to a required positive practice of one of two roles: the initiator who invited to share, and the acceptor who agreed to share. This type of positive practice led to decreases in the nonsharing behaviors, with concomitant increases in sharing behaviors.

Overcorrection has also been used in teaching correct spelling to children in elementary and junior high levels (Foxx and Jones, 1978). The children were required to correctly spell the misspelled words along with giving a dictionary definition of those words in five sentences. Studies of this kind have shown that errors of spelling can be decreased dramatically.

Overcorrection or its components have rarely been used in the clinical speech and language work. A study by Matson, Esveldt-Dawson, and O'Donnell (1979) illustrates the potential of this technique in treating certain language disorders. An elective mute boy was required to write the words he refused to speak, ten times each. As a result, the boy's speaking behavior was reinstated. It is possible that clinicians who face unruly or disruptive behaviors that alter the treatment setting can apply this technique by asking children to not only restore the situation to its original shape but also vastly improve it. A specified desirable behavior may be overpracticed.

Additional Effects of Punishment

The primary effect of the punishing stimulus is to decrease the behavior upon which it was made contingent. However, research has demonstrated that punishment may have several additional effects. Regardless of whether they were "intended" or programmed, they must be considered a part of the punishment effect. Such effects are sometimes referred to as side effects, but the term additional effects is preferred here (Matson and DiLorenzo, 1984). The term side effects suggests that we do not understand them. But in a well planned behavioral program, one should carefully analyze all effects of a contingency. The additional effects of punishment may be desirable or undesirable. The major additional effects will be summarized and procedures to control or enhance them will be described.

Undesirable Effects of Punishment

Some of the additional effects of punishment can be considered undesirable from the standpoint of the client, society, or both. Such effects are often described as negative side effects. These undesirable additional effects must be eliminated or minimized before the entire treatment program can be considered effective.

Emotional Reactions. Punishing stimuli can create some undesirable emotional reactions in the person receiving punishment. Most of the intense emotional responses have been noted with electric shock. However, any punishing stimulus can evoke negative emotional responses such as crying, whining, fear, and tantrum behaviors. Occasionally, even a firm verbal "no" can evoke certain emotional reactions in some children. If these reactions persist, it is difficult to go on with clinical training.

In clinical speech and language training, verbal punishers have been used frequently. Most clinicians tend to say "no" or "wrong" when incorrect responses are produced by their clients. Studies have generally not reported strong emotional reactions due to this type of punishing contingency. It is unlikely that an appropriate use of verbal punishing contingency would result in disruptive emotional reactions. In fact, most clients would expect the clinician to say "no" or "wrong" when their responses are not correct. Often, when the clinician fails to punish the wrong response, the client may pause and hesitate because of a lack of specific feedback. Most clients may not learn efficiently unless they receive differential feedback on the correctness of their responses.

Aggression. There is some laboratory evidence that those who are punished may show aggressive behaviors. On the basis of laboratory research, two types of aggressive behaviors have been described: elicited and operant (Azrin and Holz, 1966). Elicited aggression is directed against any object or person that simply happens to be around when punishment is delivered. It is not directed against the person punishing, and hence it does not seek to eliminate punishment. In laboratory experiments, animals receiving shocks have fought with each other or have attacked inanimate objects (Houten,

1983). However, elicited aggression itself is susceptible to punishment; such aggressive acts were effectively reduced by contingent punishment. Not many clinical studies have reported elicited aggression, but anecdotally, a child may kick the furniture or stamp the feet when told "no." A child punished during homework may throw the pencil on the ground.

Operant aggression, on the other hand, is directed against the source of punishment. Such aggressive acts could lead to a reduction in punishment. Clients who have been punished may throw objects at the clinician. In some cases, retarded and autistic subjects have tried to bite or scratch therapists administering punishment (Newsom, Favell, and Rincover, 1983).

Studies on the behavioral treatment of communicative disorders have not reported elicited or operant aggression of a serious nature. Again, an appropriately designed and managed punishment program need not lead to aggressive behaviors. This may be especially true when punishment is combined with positive reinforcement for desirable behaviors.

Escape and Avoidance. In everyday situations, one of the usual reactions to punishment is an attempt to escape or avoid the punishing agent or punishing situation. A child running away from abusive parents illustrates escape, and a child who minimizes contact with the parent who typically punishes shows avoidance. The possibility has been raised that punishment might lead clients to drop out of treatment, in which case they cannot be helped. Both basic and applied research has shown that escape and avoidance behaviors are more likely when an alternative desirable behavior is not trained and the punishment intensity is very strong. When punishment is the sole treatment procedure, avoidance and escape, whenever physically possible, may be a more certain outcome.

In considering possible escape and avoidance, one must make a distinction between the punishing agent and the punishment setting. Those who are punished may avoid not only the person administering punishment but also the entire physical setting in which it is done. Any kind of stimuli associated with punishment can acquire aversive properties and thus lead to avoidance or escape.

Paradoxical Effect. As noted before, by definition, punishment is response decrement under certain contingencies. Nevertheless, in some cases, stimuli that are well known punishers have resulted in an increase in certain response rates. Obviously, those stimuli then cannot be classified as punishing. Such increases associated with well established punishing contingencies are called paradoxical effects (Azrin and Holz, 1966).

A number of factors that may lead to the paradoxical effects of punishment have been identified. First, a very mild punisher might act as a reinforcer. Mild but constant naggings and reprimands may actually facilitate responses. It is known that mild electric shocks can facilitate responses. A second factor is the correlated administration of punishment and reinforcement. If punishment is often followed by positive reinforcement, then the punishing stimulus becomes a discriminative stimulus for reinforcement. The result might be an increase in the rate of response being "punished." The third factor involves the possibility that the punished response is based upon fear or anxiety, and that the punishment reinstates that emotional response leading to response facilitation. For example, a child's crying behavior might increase under a known punishment procedure. Fourth, punishment itself may lead to a successful escape from the punishing environment. In TO, for example, a child may be sent to his or her room for a specified misbehavior, but this may be reinforcing in the sense that the child escapes the punishing situation and enters a less aversive personal room. Timeout in such cases might increase the response upon which it was made contingent. Fifth, the paradoxical effects may be in some cases due to a unique conditioning history of the individual receiving the punishment. For example, Patterson (1976) has reported that children who come from aggressive families are more likely to show increased aggressive behaviors when punished.

Applied studies have shown that electric shock, TO, overcorrection, and verbal reprimands can increase response rates in some situations. Whenever this happens, the contingency is classified as reinforcing, and the reasons for such paradoxical effects are analyzed. Essentially, the analysis focuses upon the positive reinforcer that becomes associated with punishment.

Punishment Contrast. Punishment contrast is also a phenomenon of response increase rather than decrease, but it happens in a situation where punishment is not in effect. In paradoxical effects, responses increase while still under a known punishment contingency, whereas in contrast, there is discrimination. The response rate may decrease as long as the punishing contingency is in effect, but it may increase either in the same situation or in a different situation as long as the contingency is not in effect. Punishment contrast would be evident only when the response rate increases beyond its original baseline. The increase in response rates due to punishment contrast is known to be a temporary phenomenon.

Punishment contrast has been unequivocally demonstrated in laboratory research. In applied human research, a few studies have indicated that it may occur in some cases. For example, Merbaum

(1973) found that self-injurious behaviors decreased when punished in school, but increased at home. Punishment contrast has not been systematically studied in the treatment of communicative disorders.

Response Substitution. Sometimes a decrease in a punished response may result in an increase in some other undesirable response. A punished response may have been successful in gaining certain reinforcers from others. It is possible that the same reinforcer can be obtained by another undesirable response, which may then increase. For example, an autistic child may have received staff attention by indulging in headbanging behavior. When this behavior is punished, the child may resort to scratching his or her face. This phenomenon is known as response substitution.

Response substitution has been frequently observed in autistic or profoundly retarded persons with a variety of self-stimulatory or self-injurious behaviors. Although there have been no systematic studies, speech and language clinicians might notice response substitution when certain interfering behaviors are punished. For example, when a child's excessive hand movements are reduced by punishment, disruptive leg movements might increase.

A common tactic used to control response substitution is to apply the punishing contingency to the newly emerged or increased (undesirable) behavior as well. When there are multiple undesirable behaviors or new ones emerge, for whatever reason, the punishing contingency must be applied to those behaviors simultaneously or sequentially.

Generalized Suppression. Just as the effect of a reinforcer can spread to other stimulus conditions or responses, the effects of a punishing stimulus can also spread to other situations, persons, or responses. In effect, punishment has its counterpart of stimulus and response generalization. Obviously, stimulus and response generalization of punishment effect is very desirable, and this will be discussed along with desirable additional effects of punishment. The negative side of this phenomenon is observed when a punished person shows suppression of desirable behaviors as well, or when a response punished in one situation is indeed appropriate in another situation but does not occur because of the punishment.

Fortunately, generalized suppressive effects are known to be temporary. As treatment continues, these undesirable effects usually disappear. This seems to be the case especially when desirable, alternative behaviors are reinforced while the subject is punished for some undesirable behavior (Newsom et al., 1983). Also, generalized suppression has not been as widespread a problem as it could have been in applied research. Like the effect of reinforcement, the effect of punishment has been slow to generalize to untreated settings and responses. Typically, punished responses remain suppressed in the punished situation but high in situations not associated with punishment (Newsom et al., 1983).

Imitative Punishment. It is considered possible that those who frequently use punishment as a means of controlling behaviors set an example, especially for young children. The children in turn may be more likely to use punitive and aggressive means of controlling other people at the expense of positive means. This possibility has been discussed in relation to abusive parents who, as children, may have have been excessively punished. There is no strong evidence to support this hypothesis, but it cannot be ruled out.

Research on social learning theory has demonstrated that children do learn aggressive behaviors just by watching models who exhibit aggression. In addition, specific punishment procedures may be acquired by children exposed to such procedures. A study by Gelfand and co-workers (1974) has shown that children who were punished with response cost were likely to use the same procedure with other children.

Again, imitative punishment has not been systematically studied in the context of communicative disorders. It is possible that normal, well planned use of punishment may not necessarily result in imitative punishment.

Perpetuation of Punishment. A final concern with the use of punishment is that it may perpetuate itself. Punishment affects those who receive as well as those who administer it. A person punishes another individual's behavior precisely because that behavior is aversive to him or her. Successful acts of punishment terminate aversive events. As a result, the person who punishes others is negatively reinforced. The person who has such a history of negative reinforcement may be more likely to use punishment than positive reinforcement in controlling other individuals' aversive behaviors.

Perpetuation of punishment has obvious social implications. Although it appears reasonable, the possibility has not been empirically verified. Once again, this possibility may not be high when the clients are punished for wrong responses only when they are also positively reinforced for correct responses.

The negative additional effects of punishment described so far have not posed insurmountable problems in clinical situations. There is plenty of information on the prudent use of punishment which can minimize chances of undesirable additional effects. In a later section, the most appropriate ways of using punishment will be described.

Desirable Effects

The undesirable effects of punishment are better known than the desirable additional effects. Research has suggested the possibility of at least five positive additional effects of punishment: appropriate generalization, improved social behaviors, positive emotional responding, better attending behaviors, and facilitation of learning (Newsom et al., 1983).

Appropriate Generalization. Since individual behaviors are members of larger response classes, a single response punished and suppressed may have an effect upon other responses of the same class. Also, since punishment has its antecedents, the punished response may be suppressed in the presence of similar antecedents. If these two things were to happen, we would have a very desirable additional effect of punishment. In order to suppress a variety of undesirable behaviors, the clinician may need to punish just a few responses of that class. To the extent that nontreatment situations share some stimulus similarities with the treatment setting, the behaviors may be reduced in those situations as well.

A certain degree of stimulus and response generalization of punishment is known to take place. However, appropriate generalization does not take place as often as desired. As noted earlier, the punishment effect is more often discriminated than generalized. However, there are procedures to enhance appropriate generalization. If punishment is delivered in different situations and by different clinicians during an adequate sampling of undesirable behaviors, it might be possible to promote appropriate generalization of punishment effects.

Improved Social Behaviors. When a client's aggressive, uncooperative, unsociable behaviors are reduced by punishment, there may be an increase in socially acceptable behaviors. These improved social behaviors can be considered additional desirable effects as long as they are not specifically programmed and reinforced. Several studies have shown that either during or following punishment, clients become socially more responsive. In schizophrenic, autistic, and retarded subjects, punishment of specified undesirable behaviors has resulted in more cooperation, greater sociability, better interaction with peers and staff, and generally improved behaviors. In addition, some studies have reported that punishment of self-stimulatory behaviors in autistic children can increase appropriate, unreinforced play activities (Newsom et al., 1984).

From a logical standpoint, reduction in undesirable behaviors makes it possible for clients to engage in more productive behaviors that are naturally reinforcing. When a client is not spending much time exhibiting nonproductive behaviors, opportunities for productive behaviors become more real. In order for improved social behaviors to be maintained, however, they must sooner or later come under the influence of naturally occurring or clinically programmed reinforcement contingencies.

Emotional Behaviors. An improvement in emotional responding has also been reported as an additional desirable effect of punishment. Again, most of the studies are done with autistic children, whose self-stimulatory or self-injurious behaviors were punished. As a result, the children have been reported to smile and laugh more often and to cry and whine less frequently. Some children have also been reported to be calm and relaxed following punishment.

Attending Behaviors. Most children who indulge in self-stimulatory and self-injurious behaviors pay very little attention to their surroundings. People and events fail to draw their attention. As a result, it is generally difficult to teach them adaptive behaviors or academic skills. In some punishment studies, when self-stimulatory and self-injurious behaviors were reduced by punishment, the children's attending behaviors improved. More consistent eye contact has been reported when autistic children's self-stimulatory behaviors were punished. In other studies, subsequent to punishment, some children began to pay more attention to surrounding events, people, teaching targets, and academic skill training (Newsom et al., 1983).

Facilitation of Learning. It is logical to expect that improved attending behaviors would have some beneficial effects upon learning specific tasks. Such an outcome has been reported by several investigators. Following punishment, autistic children were better able to imitate various target behaviors. In one study (Bucher and Lovaas, 1968), when an autistic child's oppositional behavior was punished, his speech imitation increased 100 percent. Possibly, suppression of undesirable behaviors removes barriers to learning more appropriate behaviors.

How to Program Punishing Contingencies

Clinical experience shows that the use of punishing contingencies cannot be totally relinquished. Many clients' interfering and undesirable behaviors have long histories. Those behaviors compete with new skills targeted for clinical training. In such situations, an exclusive use of reinforcement contingencies may be inefficient. Punishment contingencies, used properly, may not have many of the negative effects discussed earlier and in fact may speed up the clinical learning process.

An appropriate use of punishment contingencies takes careful planning, however. Punishing contingencies must be planned in such a way that they (1) minimize or eliminate the undesirable additional effects, (2) enhance desirable additional effects, and (2) increase the chances of learning specific target behaviors. Originally, Azrin and Holz described how to program punishment in their 1966 review of punishment, which has since become a classic in the literature. Only a few additional strategies have been suggested in subsequent years (Axelrod and Apsche, 1983; Matson and DiLorenzo, 1984). What follows is based upon this available research information on the most effective use of punishment.

Punish Every Instance of the Target Behavior. The behavior to be reduced must be punished on a continuous schedule, especially in the beginning stages of treatment. In some cases, punishment may have to stay on a continuous schedule throughout the training program. However, when the response has been suppressed to a very low level of frequency, an intermittent schedule may be able to keep it at that level.

It must be realized that continuous punishment of an undesirable behavior is not always possible, because the behavior may be exhibited outside the clinic and may be reinforced there. Therefore, the fact that the clinician punishes a response every time it is produced does not necessarily mean that the behavior actually comes under a continuous schedule of punishment.

Punish Responses Immediately. Any delay in the introduction of the punishing stimulus weakens the effect. The stimulus must be delivered swiftly and immediately. When a wrong response is observed, some clinicians tend to hesitate in delivering the punishing stimulus. They may wait for a few seconds before saying "no" or "stop." This hesitation and delay in delivering the punishing stimulus is not desirable.

Punish the Earliest Sign of the Initial Response of a Chain. Most responses are actually chains of several different responses. For example, a child sitting in the living room decides to swim for a while in the family swimming pool at a wrong time. Announcing his or her plan of action, the child might leave the living room, walk toward the bedroom, grab the swim trunks, begin to undress, change into the swimming trunks, come out of the room, walk toward the patio door, open it, walk toward the swimming pool, and get ready to jump into the pool. This shows that what is normally considered to be a single integrated act of "going to swim" is actually a chain of responses. Each response in the chain takes the child closer to the terminal response of swimming (which can also be broken down into its component parts). A parent wishing to stop this behavior can intervene at various stages in the sequence. The parent may say "no swimming" just before the child is ready to jump into the pool, or as soon as the plan of action is announced, and of course any time in between. The most effective time to say "no" is when the child talks about swimming and begins to leave the living room. Saying "no" just before the child is about to jump into the pool is probably least effective.

In clinical sessions, it is important to recognize the sequence of responses that constitute target behaviors so that the earliest indication of the first element of the chain of response can be punished. In treating a /w/ for /r/ substitution, for example, the clinician can either let the child fully say "wadio" and then punish, or punish as soon as the child begins to round his lips for the production of the initial /w/ sound.

In the treatment of fluency disorders, it is very important to punish the earliest responses of the chain of stuttering. It is more effective to say "no" or "stop" as soon as the clinician hears the initial repetition of the sound than to wait until the person has completed the stuttered response (t-t-t-t-time). At times, punishment can be delivered even before the stuttered word becomes audible. In some cases, certain articulatory postures precede the actual stuttered production of a word, and punishment can be delivered at this point. In certain treatment programs, stutterers are taught to first inhale, then exhale slightly, and start phonation in a gentle, soft manner. If the stutterer forgets to inhale just before saying a word, he or she should be punished immediately rather than when the word is spoken. Similarly, the instant the exhalation is missed before phonation is started, the stutterer must be punished.

Catching a response in its earliest stage requires that the clinician pay very close attention to client behaviors and determine the beginning characteristics of target responses.

Punish with the Maximum Stimulus Intensity. It is well known that a gradual increase in the intensity of the punishing stimulus can reduce the effect of the contingency. This might happen because of the potential adaptation to the punishing stimulus. The intensity of the verbal "no," for example, must be as high as it should be from the very beginning, and should not be increased in gradual steps. If physical stimulus such as noise is used, it should be introduced at the maximum strength. Parents who gradually increase the intensity of their verbal reprimands find that reprimands of progressively higher intensity are required to draw their children's attention. Eventually, parents may find out that even loud shouts are ineffective.

Minimize Chances for Escape. When a response comes under punishing contingency, as far as possible there should be no possibility of escape. Under TO, for example, a crying child should not be able to leave the therapy room and go to the parent(s). When verbal "no" is made contingent on wrong responses, the child should not have a chance to crawl under the table or leave the therapy setting.

Minimize the Duration of Punishment. The duration of punishment should be as brief as it can be. Prolonged use of punishment suggests either that the punishing stimulus is not strong or is not effective at all, or that some of the alternative procedures (such as reinforcement of desirable behaviors) are not used properly. For example, TO should be very brief.

Dissociate the Punishing Stimulus from Reinforcement. The clinician must make sure that the delivery of punishment does not follow the delivery of reinforcers. The clinician might say "no" but immediately smile and touch the child. A parent who punishes a child might feel guilty and immediately hug the child or give something special. In such cases, punishment leads to positive reinforcement and therefore it becomes a discriminative stimulus for undesirable responses. As a result, what is thought to be a punishing stimulus might actually increase the response for which it has been programmed. On the other hand, if one makes sure that reinforcement of any kind does not follow punishing stimuli, then those stimuli will become discriminative of extinction (lack of reinforcement). In essence, the punishing stimulus should also be a discriminative stimulus for extinction, not reinforcement.

Eliminate Reinforcers for Undesirable Behaviors. This is not the same as the discriminative value of punishment just described. As noted, punishment becomes discriminative of reinforcement when a reinforcer is delivered soon after the delivery of a punishing stimulus. However, an undesirable response may be directly reinforced in one situation but punished in other situations and perhaps by other persons. In such cases, punishment may not be successful.

A response under extinction is punished more easily than the one being reinforced. For example, the clinician might be punishing gestures and vocal grunts in a nonverbal child, while reinforcing more appropriate verbal responses. However, if those gestures and grunts continue to receive reinforcement at home and at other places, the punishment programmed by the clinician may not be very effective. Clinicians might also reinforce faulty articulations or stutterings while talking with the client after the session is over. In natural settings, one of the parents may be reinforcing an undesirable behavior while the other is trying to reduce it. In programming punishment, such reinforcers must be eliminated or minimized. In the treatment settings, the clinician must insist upon the production of target behaviors from the beginning to the end of interactions, not just during the therapy time.

Reinforce an Alternative, Desirable Response. While punishing undesirable responses, the clinician must always make sure that a desirable alternative has been clearly identified to the client, and its occurrences are positively reinforced. When the client can gain access to reinforcers through desirable behaviors, punished undesirable behaviors decline fast. In this case, the undesirable behaviors have nothing to lose. Many experts believe that the key to a successful punishment contingency that does not generate undesirable side effects is to reinforce an alternative response.

Laboratory studies have shown that multiple contingencies are more effective than a single contingency. In fact, when the clinician tries to minimize reinforcement for undesirable behaviors and avoid the discriminative reinforcement value of punishment, multiple contingencies are used. An addition of a positive reinforcer for an alternative response will make the entire arrangement much more powerful.

It is probably not very useful, nor is it ethically justifiable, to exclusively punish a faulty articulation of /s/ when the client does not have a more appropriate behavior in the repertoire. When better productions of the /s/ are not targeted for reinforcement, "punishment" of the error response is not likely to be effective. It may generate undesirable side effects.

The principle should be applied in controlling nonspeech target behaviors as well. If the clinician punishes a client for looking away from stimulus materials, then reinforcers must be given for looking at the relevant stimuli. If off-seat behaviors are punished, in-seat behaviors must be reinforced.

Generally speaking, it is desirable to keep the ratio between punishment and reinforcement in favor of reinforcement. If the amount of punishment exceeds the amount of reinforcement, then a likely result is loss of motivation or the emergence of an undesirable effect.

SUMMARY

An important task of the clinician is to decrease certain undesirable behaviors exhibited by clients. Extinction and punishment are two procedures to be used in decreasing response rates.

In extinction, reinforcers of responses are simply withdrawn. With a possible initial increase, the response rate eventually decreases as a result of this procedure.

A response that has been reinforced intermittently, with large amounts of reinforcement, over a long period of time, and with no prior history of extinction, is the most difficult to extinguish.

In order to be effective, a response under extinction should not be reinforced. It is best to combine extinction for undesirable behaviors with reinforcement for desirable behaviors.

Extinction is not a method of choice for aggressive and self-injurious behaviors.

Punishment consists of empirically verified procedures that when made contingent on responses decrease the rate of that response.

Whether a stimulus is defined as punishing or not depends upon the response rate, and not upon subjective evaluations and prior opinions about that stimulus.

There are at least three different types of punishment. In Type I, presentation of a stimulus contingent upon a response results in the decreased rate of that response. In Type II, reinforcers or reinforcing states of affairs are terminated contingent upon a response, and as a result there is a decrease in that response. In Type III, response reduction is achieved by making a certain amount of work and effort contingent upon that response.

The effect of punishment is a function of several variables. It depends upon such factors as the intensity of the stimulus, the schedule of delivery, motivation or reinforcement for the punished response, discriminative value of the punishing stimulus, availability of an alternative, reinforced responses, and so on.

Punishment may induce certain undesirable effects. These include emotional reactions, aggression, escape and avoidance, paradoxical effects, punishment contrast, response substitution, generalized suppression, imitative punishment, and perpetuation of punishment.

Some of the desirable additional effects of punishment include appropriate generalization, improved social behaviors, improved emotional behaviors, attending behaviors, and facilitation of learning.

A carefully planned and executed program of punishment will minimize or eliminate the undesirable effects while enhancing the desirable ones. Such a punishment program is needed in most treatment sessions.

In order to be effective, the punishing stimulus must be delivered immediately, at the earliest sign of the response to be punished, and at maximum intensity. The punishing stimulus should not be discriminative of reinforcement, but rather, extinction. The schedule should be continuous, at least initially, and the intensity should not be increased gradually. Reinforcement for punished responses must be eliminated or reduced. An alternative desirable response must always be reinforced. The punishment duration should be brief, and in any given treatment setting, the amount of reinforcement should exceed that of punishment.

STUDY GUIDE

Answer the following questions in technical language. Check your answer with the text. Rewrite your answers when needed.

1. Describe some of the undesirable and interfering behaviors of both child and adult clients.
2. Distinguish between undesirable and interfering behaviors.
3. What are the two major sets of techniques to decrease behaviors?
4. Define extinction and give some examples.
5. What are the four factors that affect extinction?
6. How can you identify reinforcers to be withheld in extinction?
7. What is the best way of extinguishing a response? What other contingency would you combine with extinction, and how?
8. What are the negative additional effects of extinction?
9. What are the limitations of extinction?
10. What kinds of behaviors are not suitable for extinction?
11. Specify a general definition of punishment.
12. How many types of punishment were described in the text?
13. What is Type I punishment?
14. What kinds of stimuli have been used in Type I punishment?
15. What type of punishment is timeout?
16. Define timeout.
17. Distinguish between different types of timeout.

18. Which type of timeout is most suitable for reducing undesirable behaviors in clinical speech-language work?
19. What is the most effective way of using timeout?
20. Define response cost, and distinguish it from timeout.
21. When is it not possible to use response cost?
22. What is the best way of using response cost?
23. Describe the three components of overcorrection.
24. List, define, and describe all kinds of undesirable effects of punishment that were discussed in the text. Give your own examples.
25. What are the two kinds of aggression described under undesirable effects of punishment?
26. Specify five factors that may be responsible for increases in a response that has been "punished" by known punishers.
27. Distinguish between punishment contrast and paradoxical effects.
28. What do we mean when we say that in punishment contrast, there is discrimination?
29. What is the common tactic of handling response substitution?
30. What kinds of populations have most frequently shown response substitution?
31. What is the role of negative reinforcement in the perpetuation of punishment?
32. Are there many studies documenting undesirable effects of punishment in communicative disorders?
33. List, define, and describe all kinds of desirable effects that were discussed in the text. Give examples from your own experience.
34. Does the punishment effect generalize easily?
35. Compare and contrast generalization and discrimination in relation to the punishment effect.
36. What is the recommended way of programming punishing contingencies? List and describe all of the recommended strategies.
37. Describe the best way of punishing a chained response.
38. What is the best schedule of punishment in the early stages of training?
39. What is the effect of delayed punishment?
40. What do you do in order to avoid potential adaptation to the punishing stimulus?
41. How does a punishing stimulus acquire discriminative stimulus value (signaling reinforcement)?
42. Distinguish between dissociating the punishing stimulus from reinforcement and eliminating the reinforcer for undesirable behaviors.

43. What is a potential mistake committed by the clinician when the session is over?
44. Specify the importance of reinforcing alternative, desirable behaviors in implementing punishment procedures.
45. What are the potential effects of not keeping the reinforcement-punishment ratio in favor of reinforcement?
46. Justify the need for punishment procedures in clinical speech and language services.
47. Compare and contrast popular concepts and the technical definition of punishment.
48. What are the problems with the social or legal use of punishment procedures?

REFERENCES

Axelrod, S., and Apsche, J. (Eds.) (1983). *The effects of punishment on human behavior.* New York: Academic Press.

Azrin, N. H., and Holz, W. C. (1966). Punishment. In W. K. Honig (Ed.), *Operant behavior: Areas of research and application.* New York: Appleton-Century-Crofts.

Barton, E. S., and Osborne, J. G. (1978). The development of classroom sharing by a teacher using positive practice. *Behavior Modification, 2,* 231–250.

Brantner, J. P., and Doherty, M. A. (1983). A review of timeout: A conceptual and methodological analysis. In J. Aspche and S. Axelrod (Eds.), *The effects of punishment on human behavior* (pp. 87–132). New York: Academic Press.

Bucher, B., and Lovaas, I. O. (1968). Use of aversive stimulation in behavior modification. In M. R. Jones (Ed.), *Miami symposium on the prediction of behavior, 1967: Aversive stimulation.* Coral Gables, FL: University of Miami Press.

Costello, J. M. (1975). The establishment of fluency with timeout procedures: Three case studies. *Journal of Speech and Hearing Disorders, 40,* 216–231.

Ferster, C. B., Culbertson, S., and Boren, M. C. P. (1975). *Behavior principles* (2nd ed.). Englewood Cliffs, NJ: Prentice-Hall.

Ferster, C. B., and Skinner, B. F. (1957). *Schedules of reinforcement.* New York: Appleton-Century-Crofts.

Foxx, R. M., and Bechtel, D. R. (1983). Overcorrection: A review and analysis. In S. Axelrod and J. Apsche (Eds.), *The effects of punishment on human behavior* (pp. 133–220). New York: Academic Press.

Foxx, R. M., and Jones, J. R. (1978). A remediation program for increasing the spelling achievement of elementary and junior high school students. *Behavior Modification, 2,* 211–230.

Gelfand, D. M., Hartmann, D. P., Lamb, A. K., Smith, C. L., Mahan, M. A., and Paul, S. C. (1974). The effects of adult models and described alternatives on children's choice of behavior management techniques. *Child Development, 45,* 585–593.

Halvorson, J. (1971). The effect on stuttering frequency of pairing punishment (response cost) with reinforcement. *Journal of Speech and Hearing Research, 14,* 356–364.

Hegde, M. N. (1985). Treatment of fluency disorders: State of the art. In J. M. Costello (Ed.), *Speech disorders in adults: Recent advances* (pp.155–188). San Diego: College-Hill Press.

Hegde, M. N., and Gierut, J. (1979). The operant training and generalization of pronouns and a verb form in a language delayed child. *Journal of Communication Disorders, 12,* 23–34.

Holland, J. C., and Skinner, B. F. (1961). *The analysis of behavior.* New York: McGraw-Hill.

Houten, R. V. (1983). Punishment: From the animal laboratory to the applied setting. In S. Axelrod and J. Apsche (Eds.), *The effects of punishment on human behavior* (pp. 13–44). New York: Academic Press.

Ingham, R. J. (1984). *Stuttering and behavior therapy: Current status and experimental foundations.* San Diego: College-Hill Press.

James, J. E. (1981). Behavioral self-control of stuttering using time-out from speaking. *Journal of Applied Behavior Analysis, 14,* 25–37.

Kazdin, A. E. (1984). *Behavior modification in applied settings* (3rd ed.). Homewood, IL: Dorsey Press.

Martin, R. R., Khul, P., and Haroldson, S. K. (1972). An experimental treatment with two preschool children. *Journal of Speech and Hearing Research, 15,* 743–752.

Martin, R. R., St. Louis, K., Haroldson, S. K., and Hasbrouck, J. (1975). Punishment and negative reinforcement using electric shock. *Journal of Speech and Hearing Research, 18,* 478–490.

Matson, J. L., and DiLorenzo, T. M. (1984). *Punishment and its alternatives.* New York: Springer Publishing Co.

Matson, J. L., Esveldt-Dawson, K., and O'Donnell, D. (1979). Overcorrection, modeling and reinforcement procedures for reinstating speech in a mute boy. *Child Behavior Therapy, 1,* 363–371.

Merbaum, M. (1973). The modification of self-destructive behavior by a mother-therapist using aversive stimulation. *Behavior Therapy, 4,* 442–447.

Newsom, C., Favell, J. E., and Rincover, A. (1983). Side effects of punishment. In S. Axelrod and J. Apsche (Eds.), *The effects of punishment on human behavior* (pp. 285–316). New York: Academic Press.

Patterson, G. R. (1976). The aggressive child: Victim and architect of a coercive system. In E. J. Mash, L. J. Hamerlynck, and L. C. Handy (Eds.), *Behavior modification and families* (pp. 267–316). New York: Brunner/Mazel.

Pazulinec, R., Meyerrose, M., and Sajwaj, T. (1983). Punishment via response cost. In S. Axelrod and J. Apsche (Eds.), *The effects of punishment on human behavior* (pp. 71–86). New York: Academic Press.

Siegel, G. M. (1970). Punishment, stuttering, and disfluency. *Journal of Speech and Hearing Research, 13,* 677–714.

Sundel, M., and Sundel, S. S. (1975). *Behavior modification in the human services.* New York: Wiley.

Whaley, D. L., and Malott, R. W. (1971). *Elementary principles of behavior.* Englewood Cliffs, NJ: Prentice-Hall.

Chapter 9

Treatment Programs II: How to Write, Modify, and Execute Them

So far, most of the basic principles and procedures of treatment have been discussed. Procedures to increase as well as decrease target behaviors have been discussed. Response maintenance strategies have also been considered.

In Chapter 9, the following will be described:

- How to write comprehensive treatment programs for individual clients with a variety of communicative disorders
- Follow-up and booster treatment
- How to modify treatment programs to suit individual clients
- Factors determining sequences of treatment

In Chapter 5, a basic treatment program was presented. In the subsequent chapters, other aspects of the program were described. The techniques described so far should make it possible to establish certain target behaviors and get them generalized to, and maintained in, everyday situations. In this final chapter, some advanced features of the program will be discussed, and the information presented in all of the previous chapters will be integrated into a single treatment perspective. The main focus of this chapter will be on how to write comprehensive treatment programs for individual clients. The related issue of how to modify a written program in the light of clinical data will be described, along with follow-up and booster treatment procedures.

HOW TO WRITE TREATMENT PROGRAMS

Careful planning is necessary before treatment is started. It is better to have a total treatment perspective from the very beginning.

There are two approaches to treatment planning. A more traditional approach involves writing what are often referred to as "lesson plans." Lesson plans typically suggest short term objectives and procedures. They are at best sketchy. They only hint at what may be done during the current week or two weeks. Often they pertain to single sessions. Not being comprehensive, lesson plans do not give a total picture of the treatment planned for the client. The clinician writing lesson plans may not have a long-range plan or perspective. This piecemeal approach to treatment planning is not a desirable strategy.

An alternative to lesson plans is to write a comprehensive treatment program for the client at the very outset. The treatment program should include (1) the target behaviors that need to be trained, (2) a tentative sequence in which they will be trained, (3) complete treatment and probe procedures, (4) a maintenance program, (5) various criteria that will suggest movement throughout the training stages and sequences, and (6) record keeping, follow-up, and booster treatment procedures.

Writing a comprehensive treatment program takes extra planning time before treatment is initiated. However, this time will have been well spent, since the clinician does not have to think of target behaviors and treatment procedures on a weekly basis. Such planning might minimize some clinician anxieties due to uncertainties about what to do this week or next week. The program can be written in such a way that it can be easily modified to suit the needs of individual clients.

What follows is an outline of a treatment program. Much of the information needed to develop a training program has been presented in the previous chapters. For example, selection and definition of target behaviors, tentative training sequence, treatment and probe procedures, maintenance program, and criteria of movement throughout the treatment and probe sequences have been described before, as have the procedures of record keeping, follow-up, and booster treatment. Therefore, these aspects of the program will not be elaborated in the outline. The outline is intended as a checklist of areas that should be covered by a comprehensive treatment plan. It contains definitions of key terms and most of the procedures that should be specified in a treatment program.

The treatment program is written in a narrative form, much like an assessment report. With the format presented here, it should be possible to write comprehensive treatment programs for a variety of clients exhibiting different kinds of communicative disorders.

AN OUTLINE OF A GENERAL TREATMENT PROGRAM

Assess the Client's Communicative Behaviors

As soon as a need for clinical treatment has been identified for a given client, a thorough assessment of that client's speech and language behaviors is undertaken. Assessment is measurement of the client's relevant behaviors.

Take a case history.

Take reliable, valid speech and language samples. Whenever possible, take samples from the client's natural environment. Generally, repeated samples will help establish reliability.

Make a brief assessment of general and speech related motor behaviors. Make a more detailed assessment if there is evidence of neuromotor involvement, and then refer to a neurologist.

Screen hearing; refer to an audiologist when a referral is warranted.

If you wish to administer standardized tests, select those that directly sample observable speech and language behaviors instead of unobservable psychological, neurological, or cognitive processes presumed to underlie those behaviors. Keep in perspective the limitations of standardized tests, and treat all test results as tentative.

Develop and use client-specific measurement procedures. Do not hesitate to replace standardized tests with such procedures, along with carefully planned baselines.

Analyze the assessment data: the length of typical utterance (the statistical mode), the longest and shortest utterances, mean length of utterances, missing grammatic features based on obligatory contexts, frequency with which various grammatic (and semantic and pragmatic) structures are used by the client, the number and frequency of response classes produced, types of sentences used and not used, types and amounts of dysfluencies and associated motor behaviors, articulation of speech sounds at different levels of response complexity; and voice characteristics and deviations can all be specified.

Make sure the summarized client behaviors are objective and measurable. Avoid inferred, unmeasurable processes and subjective statements not backed up by objective data.

Select Target Behaviors for Training

After an assessment is made, the clinician's next task is to select target behaviors for the client. Target behaviors are empirical response classes that when modified will reduce or eliminate the disorder under consideration. Both short term and long term target behaviors must be identified. Short term target behaviors can be arbitrarily defined as those that can be trained in two to three months, whereas long term targets include most of the communicative behaviors that a given client needs to learn.

Consider the issues: What are communicative behaviors, and what behaviors are to be trained? Consider normative versus the client-specific strategies: norms and normative sequences; relevancy, usefulness, and maintenance considerations; empirically based response classes; responses that are modifiable; and so on. Should the target behaviors be trained in their normative sequence if known, or should the order depend upon clinical evidence?

Establish the Baselines of Target Behaviors

Once the target behaviors are selected, the next step is to establish the baselines of those behaviors. Baselines are reliable response measures in the absence of the planned treatment variables. Because of the limitations of the traditional assessment data, baselines are critical in establishing clinician accountability and treatment effectiveness.

Prepare the stimulus materials for evoking responses during baseline trials or periods. In many cases, the same stimuli can be used to train and probe.

Write up sentences, phrases, and words that will serve as target behaviors. Write specific questions designed to evoke the target responses.

If the client is capable of connected speech, establish baselines in conversational speech.

Establish baselines in all relevant response modes (modeled, evoked, conversational, oral reading).

When necessary, use the discrete trial procedure. A trial is a sequence of events: presenting a stimulus, asking a question, modeling a response when planned, waiting for a response (few seconds), recording the response, and moving or removing the stimulus. The sequence is then repeated with an intertrial interval of 3 to 4 seconds. Use a two trial (evoked and modeled) procedure.

During the baseline sessions, reinforce the client on a noncontingent basis.

Design a recording sheet on which every response is recorded as either correct, incorrect, or absent, using separate symbols. Have separate recording sheets for baseline, training, and probe sessions.

Whenever possible, obtain measures of communicative behaviors tape recorded in the client's home and other extraclinical situations.

Calculate the percentages of correct and incorrect productions of target responses.

Design a Flexible Therapeutic Environment

A therapeutic environment is a relatively controlled and isolated situation in which the treatment variables are applied in order to initially establish the target behaviors.

The initial therapeutic setup is a controlled environment in which the stimuli and opportunities for target behaviors are provided at full strength, whereas those for undesirable behaviors are minimized or eliminated.

However, the setup should be flexible so that during the latter stages of training, generalization can be enhanced and maintenance programs instituted by fading the difference between treatment and natural settings.

Plan and Write a Detailed Treatment Program

A treatment program spells out in detail what the client will be required to do, what the clinician will do, and how the two will interact. Ideally, the program is written up as soon as the baselines are established and before the treatment is initiated. Sometimes this may not be possible, as the clinician may wish to informally experiment with a few procedures in the first few sessions. The program should be written up as soon as possible, and should include the following: Identification data (name, address, and so on), a brief background statement, summary of assessment data, and the purposes of treatment.

The treatment program is written so that it can answer the following questions in a narrative form:

What are the target behaviors?

What are the evoked and modeled training trials? Stimulus presentation, evoking question, modeling of the correct response, time allowed to respond, reinforcement for correct responses, punishment for incorrect responses, recording procedure, and moving or removing the stimulus item should be specified. Evoked trials on which modeling is not used are similarly described.

What are correct responses? Will you accept variations? How are they scored and recorded?

What are the typical incorrect responses given by the client? How are they scored and recorded?

What are the reinforcing and punishing consequences? The types of reinforcing stimuli and punishment must be specified.

What are the schedules on which the consequences will be delivered? Initially, the reinforcers are delivered on a continuous schedule, and when the target behaviors show some significant increases (roughly a 50 percent increase above the baseline) an intermittent schedule is used. Starting with an FR2, the ratio is stretched in gradual steps.

When do you shift from modeling to evoked trials? When the discrete trials procedure is used, training starts with modeled trials, but when the client is able to imitate reliably, evoked trials are introduced. In many cases, five consecutively correct imitated responses can be sufficient to discontinue modeling.

When do you go back to modeling? Modeling is reinstated when the client gives wrong responses on two consecutive evoked trials presented soon after the termination of modeling. Subsequently, the clinician can be more flexible: Up to five incorrect responses may be accepted.

When do you reinstate evoked trials? Every time five consecutively correct imitated responses are obtained, evoked trials are presented.

What are the training criteria? There can be different training criteria, depending upon the level of training and response topography. When discrete trials are used, the criterion is usually defined in terms of the number of correct responses on a set of trials. Typically, a 90 percent correct response rate, based at least on 20 trials, is a criterion used in the initial stages of training. When discrete sentences or phrases are trained (as in language therapy), ten consecutively correct responses on a given sentence or phrase can be the initial criterion. In the treatment of fluency and voice, a 98 percent accuracy may be appropriate at all levels of treatment.

When do you probe? A probe is a procedure designed to assess generalization or maintenance of clinically trained behaviors. Probes can be administered at the completion of a training stage. When target responses are trained to a criterion at the level of single words, a probe can be administered to see if the behaviors generalize. Successive probes can be administered when target behaviors attain the training criterion at the level of phrases, sentences, or conversational speech. In the treatment of language disorders, probes can be administered after four to six stimulus items have been trained.

What is the probe criterion? The probe criterion is usually a 90 percent correct response rate on probe items. In some cases, such as stuttering, a 98 percent fluency rate may be required.

What kind of probe procedure will be used? Intermixed probes are used in the early stages, pure probes in the final stages. Responses given to the probe items are not reinforced.

What do you do when the probe criterion is not met? Any time a probe criterion is not met, the training is reinstated. The response topography or level that did not meet the probe criterion is trained again.

What is the dismissal criterion? Clients are dismissed when they meet the final dismissal criterion, which is also a probe criterion. The client can be dismissed from the continuous treatment program when responses meet at least a 90 percent probe criterion in conversational speech at home and possibly in other nonclinical situations.

How do you program response maintenance? Response maintenance is possible when target behaviors have been brought under the control of natural contingencies. Describe the maintenance procedure in terms of training other people, in other environments, and the ways in which discrimination is reduced.

When and how do you follow up? Describe the follow-up procedure. Follow-up consists of periodic measurement of trained behaviors to assess their maintenance, initially at monthly (or three month) intervals, and later at biannual and annual intervals.

What about booster treatment? Certain clients need booster treatment some time following their dismissal from treatment. Any time a follow-up measure suggests a decline in the rate of target behaviors, booster treatment must be given.

A comprehensive treatment program written according to the guidelines summarized here will make it possible to move smoothly from one level of training to the other. The program can be modified as suggested by clinical data.

Execute the Treatment Program

Careful management of behavioral contingencies is the most important aspect of implementing treatment programs. While this is being done, behaviors are constantly measured to document changes. Reinforcement, punishment, and extinction contingencies are managed throughout the treatment phase. Essentially, the clinician manages two types of contingencies: those that will increase some responses, and those that will decrease others. Certain contingencies are applied to the desirable target behaviors, and certain other contingencies are applied to undesirable target behaviors.

Apply the selected contingencies to the desirable target behaviors.

1. Select potential reinforcers.
2. Deprive, if necessary.
3. Shape the desired response whenever necessary. Do not allow the intermediate responses to stabilize. Raise the criterion of reinforcement gradually, resulting in the terminal response.
4. Model the correct responses until imitative responses are produced reliably.
5. Use other stimulus control procedures such as prompting, verbal instructions, and manual guidance.
6. Fade the stimulus control in gradual steps.
7. Reinforce responses immediately. When you use primary reinforcers, make sure you also use social reinforcers.
8. Withdraw the primary reinforcer eventually. Shift to an intermittent schedule of reinforcement.
9. Whenever possible, use generalized conditioned reinforcers. Select reinforcers from the client's natural environment.
10. Train as many response exemplars as necessary to obtain an initial generalization.

Apply the selected contingencies to undesirable behaviors.

1. Define the undesirable behaviors of the client operationally.
2. Whenever possible, identify reinforcers that may be maintaining those responses.
3. Withhold the reinforcers for inappropriate behaviors (extinction).
4. Whenever possible, remove opportunities for emitting inappropriate behaviors.
5. When selected, deliver Type I punishing stimuli ("no," "wrong," and so on) promptly and response contingently.
6. Whenever appropriate, use the Type II punishment (response cost, timeout).
7. When using the response cost procedure, withdraw reinforcers response contingently.
8. When using timeout, say "stop," avoid eye contact, and "freeze" for a few seconds.
9. Always reinforce an alternative, incompatible, desirable behavior while punishing an undesirable behavior.
10. Keep the reinforcement-punishment ratio in favor of reinforcement.
11. Watch for possible undesirable additional effects of punishment.

Plan and Execute a Maintenance Program

Almost all clients need a maintenance program. The target behaviors trained in clinical situations may show some amount of generalization to natural environments. This must be measured. However, the fact that target behaviors generalized is no assurance that they will be maintained over time. Therefore, a maintenance program must be implemented.

1. Use the probe procedure throughout the training period to monitor generalization.
2. Select responses that are useful to the client.
3. Train responses in relation to a variety of stimuli.
4. Use conditioned generalized reinforcers.
5. Use intermittent schedules of reinforcement.
6. Bring observers, parents, friends, and siblings into training sessions.
7. Move therapy to natural settings during the latter stages of training.
8. Train the production of target responses in conversational speech.
9. Reinforce generalized responses.
10. Encourage parents to observe treatment sessions.
11. Train parents, teachers, siblings and others to manage the contingencies at home, school, and other places.
12. Train parents and others to create opportunities for emitting target responses.
13. Train parents in recording speech-language samples that you can use to assess generalization and maintenance.
14. When it is practical, hold informal sessions in the client's natural environment.
15. Hold booster treatment sessions whenever follow-up measures warrant them.

Keep Continuous Objective Records

Target behaviors must be measured continuously. The traditional pretests and posttests are inadequate. Continuous objective records help establish clinician accountability.

1. Before you begin to baserate, design a recording sheet and a measurement procedure.

2. Measure the frequency of desirable and undesirable responses and record them separately.
3. Record baseline, training, and probe data on separate sheets.
4. Obtain response rates in extraclinical situations.
5. Specify the measured behaviors in terms of absolute numbers as well as percentages.
6. Avoid subjective statements that are not supported by objective measures.
7. Record the occurrence of target behaviors (desirable as well as undesirable) in each session.
8. Summarize measurement-based observations at the end of each session.

Follow Up the Client

Follow-up is a procedure designed to assess response maintenance in the natural environment and across time. Responses are measured in the absence of treatment variables.

1. Before the client is dismissed, assess generalization and maintenance of all of the trained responses in as many situations and contexts as possible.
2. Schedule initial follow-up sessions in three to six month intervals and subsequently on an annual basis.
3. Use the conversational probe procedure to assess response maintenance.
4. Whenever possible, take the follow-up measures in nonclinical situations involving people not associated with treatment.

Arrange for Booster Treatment

Many clients can benefit from a booster treatment some time after they have been dismissed from the program. A few booster sessions can strengthen responses to a great extent and thus promote maintenance.

1. Whenever a follow-up measure shows a decline in the response rate, conduct booster treatment sessions. Typically, the original treatment variables are reinstated.
2. If new treatment variables are found to be necessary, do not hesitate to use them.
3. Subsequent to booster treatment sessions, follow-up sessions should be as frequent as they were to begin with.

The outline just given can be modified as necessary. It lists components of treatment programs that are common to most disorders. Whenever individual disorders or clients seem to need additional procedures, they can be easily incorporated.

HOW TO MODIFY TREATMENT PROGRAMS

A written treatment program is useful because the clinician can organize treatment according to the preplanned sequence. However, a treatment program should not be considered a set of rules that must be followed regardless of client performance. A written program is a tentative plan of action, but what exactly the clinician does throughout the sessions depends mostly upon the client performance. The program may be executed the way it was written, or the client responses may dictate changes. Very often, treatment programs need to be modified because of changing patterns of client behaviors. Every clinician ought to know when and how to modify planned treatment procedures.

A number of client-specific reasons necessitate modifications in treatment programs. Several of these reasons are unique to individual clients, but some common reasons can be identified. The distinction between treatment principles and procedures will be helpful in considering potential modifications of a treatment program. Some suggestions for program modifications follow. Each suggestion is based upon a reason that would necessitate a change.

Principles Do Not Change; Procedures Do

Most frequently, a program needs modification because a particular procedure is not working with a given client. In such cases, the clinician should analyze specific reasons for failure and make necessary changes. An important factor to keep in perspective is that changes are almost always made in procedures, not in principles. The principles of response contingency, positive and negative reinforcement, extinction, punishment, discrimination, generalization, and environmental control (maintenance) are not modified by uncontrolled clinical activity.

Most often, what fails is a treatment procedure, not the principle behind it. Since each principle can generate different treatment procedures, it is possible to modify ineffective procedures within the framework of those principles. Usually, a more effective procedure can be derived from the same principle. For example, if verbal "no" does not reduce a client's error responses, maybe timeout will.

Selected Consequences May Not Be Effective

Probably the most common problem encountered in treatment programs is that the selected response consequences do not work. The clinician might have selected what was considered a "terrific" reinforcer, but it may not increase the rate of the target response when presented contingently. The clinician might present tokens, but they may not effect expected changes in the desirable response. Undesirable target behaviors may not decrease when the consequence is a verbal "no." In situations such as these, some clinicians say that reinforcement or punishment did not work. What really happened was that the selected response consequences did not act as reinforcers or punishers, and it is no reflection on the principle of reinforcement or punishment. The modification in this case is simple: Change the particular consequence.

Before a selected consequence is abandoned, however, the clinician must make sure that it was used correctly. Were the consequences delivered response contingently? If the training stage was initial, were they used continuously? If tokens were used, were they backed up by any kind of reinforcer? A not uncommon mistake is to present plastic chips and assume that they are reinforcers. If there were no mistakes in the use of the selected consequences, then the clinician must select new consequences. In the case of tokens, different backups must be found. If verbal stimuli such as "good" and "excellent" have not been effective, perhaps primary reinforcers or a well backed up token system will be effective. If stimuli of the Type I punishment class have not been effective, maybe response cost should be tried.

In the management of reinforcing and punishing consequences, the clinician should always adhere to the empirical definitions of reinforcers, punishers, and so on. An event is a reinforcer or punisher only after its effects upon a response rate have been established. Within this philosophy, one cannot complain about "ineffective reinforcers or punishers," which is a contradiction in terms. One can only talk about not having found a reinforcer or punisher, which means that the clinician should search for the consequences that will act as such.

Individual Histories Necessitate Changes

Treatment programs that cannot be modified to suit individual behavioral histories are not very useful to clinicians. In fact, the most important need to modify a treatment program is the unique history of an individual client. Even the possibility that certain consequences may not be effective with given clients is often a function of the individual history. As noted in earlier chapters, a child who is nonverbal, for example, may not react to verbal praise in the same way a highly verbal client does.

It is well known that what is reinforcing to one client may not be reinforcing to another. For the same client, what is reinforcing at one time may not be reinforcing at other times. Punishing events may also vary accordingly. Some clients generalize relatively easily, whereas others do not. The specific factors responsible for such individual differences may not be fully understood, but the fact that multiple procedures must be used to achieve the same goals in different clients and at different times in the same clients is very clear.

Stimulus Properties and Stimulus Control May Require Changes

It may be recalled that antecedents of target behaviors are a significant part of governing contingencies. Defective antecedents may fail to evoke responses. Pictorial and other stimulus material selected for training may be ambiguous or poor representations of real stimulus events. Poorly drawn pictures may be able to evoke the correct naming responses from a client with adequate verbal skills, but not necessarily from a language handicapped child.

The questions designed to evoke answers from the client may not be direct. In training the regular past tense inflection, for example, the clinician may have to first state what is happening in the picture and then ask what happened yesterday ("Today the man is painting; yesterday he did the same; what did he do yesterday?"). While training the present progressive, the clinician may not be able to evoke the *ing* by simply asking the client to "tell something about the picture." The question may have to be more specific, as "what is the boy doing?" Writing questions for evoking a number of grammatical features requires some thought.

In some forms of stuttering treatment, the clinician initially evokes single word or short phrase responses. This strategy may be needed in the treatment of voice disorders also. How to ask questions that restrict answers to one or two words also needs some prior planning.

When treatment is shifted from one stage to the next, the discriminative stimulus control may be lost. For example, a response that has come under the control of a modeling stimulus may be adversely affected when modeling is discontinued. Whenever loss of discriminative stimulus control seems to be the problem, the stimulus must be faded in gradual steps. If all of the *ing* responses were trained with the verbal antecedent "What is the boy doing?", then other antecedents may fail to control that response.

Response Topographies May Have to Be Changed

Another reason for modifying treatment programs is the changing nature of response properties. Verbal behavior typically consists of complex chains, the elements of which are continuously variable. As noted in earlier chapters, target behaviors can be trained at various levels of response complexity. Clients may fail to learn when a wrong level of response topography has been selected for training. In such cases, there may be nothing wrong with the contingencies used by the clinician.

The clinician who began training a certain phoneme at the phrase level might find that the correct responses are not produced frequently enough to keep the reinforcement-punishment ratio in favor of the former. Then, the response topography must be changed. The assumption is that the initial topography selected for training was not appropriate ("too difficult for the client"). Perhaps the client needs training at the level of single words.

In training grammatic features, one might initially select a sentence form, but the client may not show systematic increases in that behavior. Assuming that other procedures were correctly used, the clinician at this point might consider training the feature in the context of single words or two word phrases.

Treatment of fluency disorders also requires that the clinician give careful consideration to response topography. The treatment technique can be applied initially at the level of isolated words. If the treatment is started at the level of continuous speech, the target behaviors such as reduced rate or soft phonation may not be sustained by the stutterer.

Treatment of voice disorders, too, can pose similar problems. For example, the client may not be able to sustain the desirable pitch at the level of sentences, but may be able to do so when asked to produce single words or short phrases.

Some clients can learn certain target responses more easily than other targets. A guideline the clinician can use to judge this is the differential baserates of selected target behaviors. If the correct production of plural morpheme /s/ was baserated at 0 percent, and the present progressive *ing* at 37 percent, then the first behavior to be trained should be the *ing*. It is quite possible that because of the higher initial baseline, the *ing* will be learned relatively faster than the plural /s/. It must be noted, though, that there is not much experimental evidence to suggest that the amount or ease of training is a function of the initial baseline. Clinical experience shows that if the child is already producing a response to some extent, that response is then easier to train than a response that is not being produced at all.

Two or more behaviors that have similar baselines may be more or less difficult to learn. When a target behavior does not seem to increase under the training contingency, the clinician must move on to another target. It is hard to say when the clinician should stop training efforts on a given target, but it should not be done too prematurely.

The clinician should always remember that most target behaviors need to be shaped. A complex response topography can be simplified by breaking that response into smaller targets that are shaped in successive stages. Before dropping a particular target from training, one must make sure that the shaping procedure was tried. Of course, the clinician will return to that difficult target behavior at a later time.

Most programs, no matter how carefully written, will probably require some modifications during implementation. In modifying treatment programs, the single most important criterion to follow is the client's rate of reponses. If desirable responses do not increase, and undesirable responses do not decrease, then something is wrong. Perhaps the consequences were not functional. Stronger reinforcers were needed. The selected stimulus materials were not relevant. Maybe the response selected for training was not appropriate. Perhaps the response was appropriate but a shaping procedure was not used effectively. The clinician may not have found an initial response that exists in the client's repertoire. In modifying a program, such possibilities must be considered.

SEQUENCE OF TRAINING

In Chapter 5, a basic sequence of treatment was described. The description specified an initial sequence of training, probe, and progression across different target behaviors. In addition to describing what the client and the clinician will be doing, a treatment program describes movement. Both the client and the clinician behaviors move across different parameters. It means that "what to do next" is an important question for the program writer.

In this section, a few major factors that determine particular sequences of treatment will be considered. Treatment must be sequenced because of (1) response topographies, (2) response modes, (3) multiple targets, (4) generalization and maintenance, and (5) shifts in contingencies.

Sequenced Response Topographies

Final target behaviors are often complex and chained. Most clients are unable to learn them in total. Therefore, the final target behavior is almost always taught in small steps. The clinician first identifies what the client can do that is in some way related to the final target behavior. By making this occur more reliably, the clinician moves to the next response, which may be slightly more complex. In this way, the final target may be achieved. Of course, this is the well known shaping procedure. In essence, the most basic reason for sequencing treatment is varied response topography.

Sequencing response topographies is the heart of the shaping process, and shaping is one of the common elements of most, if not all, treatment programs. Generally speaking, the more difficult the task for a given client, the smaller the response topography at which the training is initiated. For example, when training is started at the level of syllables, it must move through the stages of words, phrases, sentences, and conversational speech. At each stage, the client's responses must meet a certain training criterion, probe criterion, or both. For example, when the correct production of the target phoneme in syllables reaches 90 percent correct across 20 consecutive trials, the clinician might shift training to the word level. A 90 percent correct response rate at the word level might suggest that the training be shifted to the phrase level, and so on.

Based upon response topographies, language training is similarly sequenced. A basic vocabulary training program, for example, might involve certain simple words. However, each word response may have to be broken into smaller responses such as the production of syllables. The syllables are then "put together" to form the word. Once a few words are taught, the clinician might move on to teaching phrases consisting of those words. Phrases may then be expanded into sentences. Essentially, training moves from simpler to more complex response classes involving varied response topographies.

In treating stuttering, the typical starting point is single words or short phrases. The target behaviors, such as rate reduction through syllable prolongation, inhalation and slight exhalation before phonation, gentle onset of phonation, and soft articulatory contacts are practiced and reinforced at the level of single words or short phrases. When these skills are stabilized at this level, the training may be shifted to expanded utterances. Eventually, the target behaviors are practiced in conversational speech.

Treatment of voice disorders also has sequences similar to those found in stuttering treatment. Whether it is the modification of vocal pitch, intensity, tremors, or other vocal qualities such as hoarseness, the treatment is started at a level of response topography the client can handle with some degree of success. The client may be asked to reduce tremors while saying simple words, or even while vocalizing a syllable. If the tremors are successfully controlled at this level, the training may be shifted to words or phrases, and finally to the level of conversational speech where the response topography is allowed to vary. Success at each stage, defined operationally, means that the client is ready for the next stage of higher response complexity.

Sequenced Response Modes

Different modes of responses create a need for sequencing training, because the target behaviors can be taught more easily in some modes than in others. The mode in which treatment is started may not be the terminal mode for that response. Therefore, the clinician often starts with one mode and finishes with another.

The most frequently used initial mode is imitative. The clinician models the correct response and the client tries to duplicate it. Success leads to reinforcement. When the target behavior is imitated reliably by the client, the modeling stimulus is faded. If additional discriminative stimulus is required, prompts are used, and they are also faded. Then, the training is shifted to a nonimitative response mode (evoked speech).

In some cases oral reading may be an initial response mode. In the treatment of adult stutterers, it is often easier to train the target responses in oral reading than in conversational speech. Oral reading frees the stutterer from the task of speech formulation. The client can concentrate upon production aspects of speech, such as slow rate and gentle onset. Also, topographical expansion, such as movement from the one word to the two word level, is easier in oral reading. Once the skills are practiced in the oral reading mode, the client must shift to the conversational speech mode. Thus, the sequence in this case might be oral reading and conversational speech, with topographically based sequences within each of these modes of responses.

Sequenced Multiple Targets

In earlier chapters it was noted that most clients have multiple responses missing in their repertoire. Especially in case of articulation and language disorders, multiple targets are the rule. Occasionally, a client might need training on a single phoneme such as /s/, but cases such as these are few. When multiple behaviors need to be trained, they must be sequenced.

In Chapter 5, the essential sequence involving multiple responses was described. When the first target behavior has reached an initial probe criterion, the clinician selects the next behavior for training. While the second behavior is being trained, the first behavior may be moved to the next topographic level. For instance, if the first behavior has reached the probe criterion at the single word level, it may be moved to the phrase level of training. The training on the second behavior will be initiated at the word level. In this manner, additional behaviors are newly brought under the training contingency while already trained behaviors keep advancing through sequences based upon response topography, mode, or other factors.

Theoretically, it is possible to train multiple targets in single sessions at the same level or different levels of response topography. In the beginning, however, it may be preferable to train only one behavior, or just a few. In the subsequent phases of treatment, multiple responses may be trained, each at a different topographic level. For example, the first grammatic feature selected for training may be now at the level of conversational speech mode. At this time, the second behavior may be trained at the controlled sentence level. The third behavior may be at the phrase level of training, and so on. How many target behaviors can be simultaneously handled in single sessions depends upon the client's sustained response rates and the length of sessions.

Training and Maintenance Based Sequences

Yet another factor that necessitates sequencing is the training-generalization-maintenance aspects that are involved in all treatment programs. Target behaviors are first trained to a certain probe criterion. When a behavior is trained at the highest topographic level and the conversational speech mode, some generalization of that behavior to natural settings might occur. However, after the initial training has been accomplished, a maintenance strategy needs to be implemented. Observers, parents, or siblings may be brought into the treatment sessions. The treatment setting may be changed. Informal treatment sessions may be held at the client's home, school, or occupational setting. The parents may be trained to administer probes and the treatment contingencies at home. All of these activities must be sequenced.

Some aspects of generalization and maintenance may be considered at the very outset of the treatment program. Selecting target behaviors that are likely to be emitted and reinforced in the natural environment would be an example. Most other aspects of generalization and maintenance are implemented only after a certain amount of training has been completed. Shifting training from a controlled to a more natural setting, for example, may not be productive if done at the very early stage of treatment. Furthermore, some parents may find it hard to reinforce a target that is still being shaped by the clinician. Therefore, these aspects of maintenance are better implemented at a later time when responses have been shaped and can now be reinforced by parents.

Sequenced Shifts in Contingencies

The final factor that dictates a sequence to be described here arises from the need to manage contingencies differently at different stages of treatment. The point was discussed in earlier chapters but needs reiteration here. In the beginning of treatment, the reinforcers are presented on a continuous schedule because this can speed up learning. However, in order to strengthen already learned responses, reinforcers are given on an intermittent schedule during the latter stages of treatment.

Any time an intermittent schedule is introduced, or a shift is made to a larger schedule, the response rate might drop. Whenever this happens, the clinician will have to reinstate the continuous reinforcement. The intermittent schedule introduced for the first time must not require a large number of responses or great intervals between reinforcers. When properly sequenced, contingency shifts can help maintain responses in natural environments.

CONCLUDING REMARKS

It is hoped that the nine chapters of this book can provide speech-language pathologists with some conceptual as well as methodologic bases of clinical intervention. In conclusion, it may be appropriate to summarize the clinical and philosophic assumptions of this book.

The first assumption is that a strong scientific basis is needed for a clinical profession such as that dealing with communicative disorders. Unless clinical practice is based on the concepts and methods of science, it is unlikely that we will gain public recognition as a profession and as a scientific discipline. In fact, unless we are first recognized as a scientific discipline, we may not gain much of a recognition as a clinical profession. Throughout the book, emphasis has been placed upon the view that experimental evidence should support clinical practice. There is an urgent need to expand clinical-experimental research activities in the field of communicative disorders. It is hoped that more and more clinicians will be inclined to gather experimental evidence as part of their clinical services.

Second, science and clinical activities are more similar than different. Science and clinical practice share common goals and procedures. Scientists and practitioners alike seek to analyze and control phenomena of their interests.

Third, as clinical scientist, speech-language pathologists must base procedures on experimental evidence and not on speculative reasoning. Normally, this should go without saying, but unfortunately it needs to be said. Also, clinical practice cannot be based upon mere observational data such as developmental trends. Clinical procedures must be experimentally tested under controlled clinical conditions.

Fourth, treatment programs must be client specific. A clinical science is needed that looks at an individual client's real behaviors and not statistical averages based upon group performances. The requirements of law and science both dictate that clinicians develop a philosophy of practice that treats individual behaviors as the ultimate test of the efficacy of treatment techniques. All treatment techniques should be modifiable in light of client-specific data.

Fifth, there are principles of treatment that apply across disorders of communication. From these principles, it is possible to derive procedures to treat individual clients and specific disorders.

Sixth, there is a treatment paradigm that fulfills these and other philosophic as well as methodologic requirements. Throughout this book, that paradigm, which describes environmental events and the client and clinical actions in terms of a contingency, has been enumerated. Treatment in communicative disorders involves a contingent relation between environmental events, client responses, and clinician actions. A successful clinician is able to manage this contingent relation to effect objectively measured changes in the client behaviors.

SUMMARY

In planning treatment for specific clients, either traditional lesson plans or comprehensive treatment programs can be written. The latter gives a better treatment perspective and hence is preferable.

The written treatment program should include target behaviors, treatment sequences, treatment and probe procedures, maintenance program, various criteria of "movement," record keeping, follow-up, and booster treatment procedures.

The treatment program that can be applied across disorders includes the following ten steps: (1) assessing the client's communicative behaviors; (2) selecting target behaviors, (3) establishing the baselines, (4) designing a flexible therapeutic environment, (5) planning and writing a detailed treatment program, (6) executing the treatment program, (7) planning and executing a maintenance program, (8) keeping continuous objective records, (9) following up of the client, and (10) arranging booster treatment.

Most treatment programs need to be modified in light of the client response data. However, it is the treatment procedures that are changed, not principles. The reasons for program modification include the following: (1) ineffective consequences, (2) unique individual histories, (3) inadequate stimulus control, and (4) inappropriate response topographies.

Almost all treatment programs have to be sequenced for the following reasons: (1) varied response topographies, (2) different response modes, (3) multiple targets, (4) training and maintenance considerations, and (5) contingency shifts.

Speech-language pathologists have a treatment paradigm that fulfills the legal, social, and scientific demands that are made upon the profession. Additional research within this conceptually and methodologically integrated model can be expected to help refine treatment procedures and extend their generality.

STUDY GUIDE

Answer the following questions in technical language. Check your answers with the text. Rewrite your answers when needed.

1. What are the two approaches to treatment planning?
2. Which one of those approaches was not recommended?

3. Why should you write a comprehensive treatment program at the very beginning?
4. What are the six major elements of a comprehensive treatment program?
5. List the ten steps of an outline of a general treatment program. Describe each step briefly.
6. What is assessment, as defined in this chapter?
7. What is a therapeutic environment?
8. Why should a therapeutic environment be flexible?
9. What are the major questions a treatment program should answer?
10. What would you list under "apply the selected contingencies to the desirable target behaviors"?
11. What would you list under "apply the selected contingencies to undesirable behaviors"?
12. List at least ten elements of a maintenance program.
13. How do you measure and record target behaviors?
14. What is a follow-up?
15. Do you reinforce during follow-up measurement?
16. How often do you schedule follow-ups?
17. What is booster treatment?
18. When is booster treatment necessary?
19. How is booster treatment given?
20. What are the five conditions that might necessitate program modifications?
21. What are the five reasons for sequencing training?
22. What are the clinical and philosophic assumptions of this book?

APPENDIX A

Hypothetical treatment data described in Chapter 5 are shown here, along with an illustration of the treatment data recording procedure.

Treatment Recording Sheet

Name: Tommy Logos   Clinician: Linda Verbose
Age: 6 years   Date: September 15, 1986
Disorders: Language   Session No. 4
Target behavior: Plural /s/   Reinforcement: continuous
  auxiliary is, prep., "on" past tense /d/   verbal, FR2 cereal

Target Responses   **Training Trials**

1. Cups   (a)   1 2 3 4 5 6 7 8 9 10 11 12 13 14 15 16 17 18 19 20
                    m− + + − + + + − + − + + + − + + + + e− −

         (b) 21 22 23 24 25 26 27 28 29 30 31 32 33 34 35 36 37 38 39 40
                    m+ + + + + e+ − + + − + + − + + + − + + +

         (c) 41 42 43 44 45 46 47 48 49 50 51 52 53 54 55 56 57 58 59 60
                    + + + + + + +

2. Boots (a) m+ + + + + + e− + + − + − + − + + + + − + +
         (b) + + + + + + + +

3. Hats   (a) m+ − + + − + + + + e− + + + − + + + + + +
         (b) + + + +

4. Plates (a) m+ + + + e+ + + + + − + + + + + + + + + +

5. Bats   (a) m+ − + + + + e+ + + − + + + + + + + + +

6. Ducks (a) m+ + + + e+ − + + + − + + + + + + + + + +

Note: (+) = correct; (−) = incorrect; (m) = modeled; (e) = evoked. The remaining three target behaviors were trained and recorded in the same manner. Separate recording sheets were used for each of those behaviors.

APPENDIX B

Hypothetical probe data on the first target behavior described in Chapter 5 are shown here. As suggested in the text, additional probe data on the same or other target behaviors were similiary recorded.

Probe Recording Sheet

Name: Tommy Logos	Clinician: Linda Verbose
Age: 6 years	Date:
Disorders: Language	Session No.
Target behavior: Plural /s/	Reinforcement: FR2
Procedures: Intermixed probe	

Target Responses	Correct (+)/Incorrect (−)	
1. Cups (T)	+	
2. Ships (U)	+	
3. Boots (T)	+	
4. Cats (U)	+	
5. Hats (T)	−	
6. Boats (U)	+	
7. Plates (T)	+	
9. Rabbits (U)	−	
10. Bats (T)	+	
11. Coats (U)	+	
12. Ducks (T)	+	
13. Nuts (U)	−	
14. Cups (T)	+	
15. Goats (U)	+	
16. Boots (T)	+	
17. Plants (U)	−	
18. Hats (T)	+	
19. Blocks (U)	+	
20. Plates (T)	+	
21. Lamps (U)	−	
22. Bats (T)	+	
23. Rats (U)	+	
24. Ducks (T)	+	
25. Ants (U)	+	
26. Cups (T)	+	
27. Trucks (U)	+	
28. Boots (T)	+	
29. Pots (U)	+	
30. Hats (T)	+	Percent correct: 64

NOTE: The trained (T) and untrained (U) items were alternated. The trained items were used repeatedly. The responses given only to the trained items were reinforced. The percent correct probe rate is based on the number of probe items only.

Author Index

Subject Index

A

Abstraction, 175
  in concept formation, 175–176
  in generalization and discrimination,
    175–176
Accountability, 15, 19, 27, 47, 114
Aggression in punishment, 223–224
Application of selected contingencies
  to desirable behaviors, 246
  to undesirable behaviors, 246
Assessment, 48–54, 113–114, 241
  as measurement, 52–54, 74
    four criteria of, 53–54
  traditional procedures of, 48–52
    case history, 48
    interview, 48
    language sampling, 49–50
    limitations of, 50–52
    oral-peripheral examination, 48
    test administration, 48–49
Attention
  as social reinforcer, 212
  as a result of punishment, 229
  in extinction, 212

B

Baselines, 33–40, 114–123, 242
  analysis of data, 122–123
  characteristics of, 115
  defined, 114
  deteriorating, 115
  procedures of, 116–122
  reasons for, 114–115
  reinforcement during, 121–122
Biofeedback, 89
Booster treatment, 201–203

C

Client-specific strategy, 64–67
  considerations in, 66–67

in the client assessment, 241
Clinical practice, contrasted with science,
  24–26
Clinicians
  as critical consumers of research, 28, 43
  two basic tasks of, 77–78, 107
Conditioned reinforcers, 83–85
Consequences
  as clinician reactions, 13
  to control responses, 77–108
Contingencies, 6–7, 16
  as treatment variables, 77–108
  defined, 6
  genetic, 6–7
  two kinds of, 6–7
    defined, 7
    environmental, 6–7, 16
    genetic and neurophysiological, 6–7
  three variables of, 7
Contingency management, 127–128,
  245–247, 258
Control group, 29
Criteria. See *Modeling; Probe;* and
  Training.

D

Decreasing undesirable behaviors,
  209–259. See also *Extinction;*
  Punishment.
Definitions of target behaviors, 67–72, 74
  constituent definitions, 68, 74
    examples of, 68–69
  operational definitions, 68–74
    examples of, 69–72
    five criteria of, 72
    limitations of, 73
Determinism, 20
Diagnosis
  in medicine, 3–4
  in communicative disorders, 3
Discrete trials, 120–121, 126, 130–139
  baseline trials, 120–121, 143
  defined, 120